COURAGE IN
HEALTHCARE

Sara Miller McCune founded SAGE Publishing in 1965 to support the dissemination of usable knowledge and educate a global community. SAGE publishes more than 1000 journals and over 800 new books each year, spanning a wide range of subject areas. Our growing selection of library products includes archives, data, case studies and video. SAGE remains majority owned by our founder and after her lifetime will become owned by a charitable trust that secures the company's continued independence.

Los Angeles | London | New Delhi | Singapore | Washington DC | Melbourne

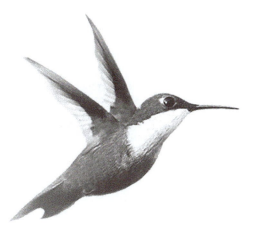

SHIBLEY RAHMAN
REBECCA MYERS

COURAGE IN HEALTHCARE

A NECESSARY VIRTUE OR WARNING SIGN?

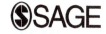

Los Angeles | London | New Delhi
Singapore | Washington DC | Melbourne

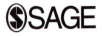

Los Angeles | London | New Delhi
Singapore | Washington DC | Melbourne

SAGE Publications Ltd
1 Oliver's Yard
55 City Road
London EC1Y 1SP

SAGE Publications Inc.
2455 Teller Road
Thousand Oaks, California 91320

SAGE Publications India Pvt Ltd
B 1/I 1 Mohan Cooperative Industrial Area
Mathura Road
New Delhi 110 044

SAGE Publications Asia-Pacific Pte Ltd
3 Church Street
#10-04 Samsung Hub
Singapore 049483

Editor: Alex Clabburn
Editorial assistant: Jade Grogan
Production editor: Rudrani Mukherjee
Copyeditor: Christine Bitten
Proofreader: Sharon Cawood
Indexer: Elske Jansen
Marketing manager: Tamara Navaratnam
Cover design: Wendy Scott
Typeset by: C&M Digitals (P) Ltd, Chennai, India
Printed in the UK

Library of Congress Control Number: 2018943847

British Library Cataloguing in Publication data

A catalogue record for this book is available from the
British Library

ISBN 978-1-5264-1358-1
ISBN 978-1-5264-1359-8 (pbk)

At SAGE we take sustainability seriously. Most of our products are printed in the UK using responsibly sourced
papers and boards. When we print overseas we ensure sustainable papers are used as measured by the PREPS
grading system. We undertake an annual audit to monitor our sustainability.

Shibley Rahman would like to dedicate this book to his mother, Hasna.

Rebecca Myers would like to dedicate this book to her father, Edward, who taught her to stand up and speak, and to her mother, Ann, who taught her to sit down and listen.

CONTENTS

LIST OF FIGURES

ABOUT THE AUTHORS

Dr Shibley Rahman is an academic physician by training, having graduated in medicine and completed his PhD at Cambridge University. He has a particular interest and specialises in wellbeing and long-term conditions. His other main focus includes employment rights and organisational culture, having completed his Master of Law and MBA both in London.

Rebecca Myers has over 30 years experience of working in and with the NHS and is an experienced board-level director, coach, OD practitioner and clinician. She has designed, facilitated and led inter and intra organisational change and leadership programmes. She recently returned to part-time practice working in community nursing, and is currently lead facilitator of Schwartz Rounds® in an acute hospital and an independent Organisational Development Specialist. Her management work has also included time within social services and the voluntary sector and her coaching career spans nearly 20 years having coached hundreds of clients including NHS Board members and senior leaders at the Department of Work and Pensions, Education and Voluntary Sector. She is a member of the British Psychological Society, The Royal College of Nursing, the Royal Society of Medicine and the Alzheimer's Society and holds a BSc in Psychology (London), an MSc in Organisational Change (Ashridge) and postgraduate qualifications in Mentoring, Coaching and Group Dynamics (Tavistock).

ACKNOWLEDGEMENTS

Firstly, we should like to thank SAGE for taking on this project, which, we feel, is an important topic for all those working in or using health and social care services.

We are both grateful for the substantial support received from the editorial and production staff at SAGE, and their guidance at several points during the process. We are especially grateful to anonymous reviewers who provided constructive feedback on the original proposal and the subsequent advice from those whose work we admire, including Jenny Rogers and Valerie Illes.

With this title, we also benefited enormously from the many people who made contributions directly or indirectly through the stories they shared with us, the research they have conducted on the subject or the examples they have shown us in our personal and professional lives. The names and details in the specific case studies have been changed to protect the anonymity of those involved. They are just some examples of the courageous work that takes place every day in social care and the National Health Service.

PUBLISHER'S ACKNOWLEDGEMENTS

On behalf of the authors, SAGE would like to thank the academic lecturers who reviewed the content of the book, helping to shape and influence it for the better.

Adriana Arcia, Columbia University

Peter Ellis, Independent Nursing and Health Care Consultant, Writer and Educator

Benny Goodman, University of Plymouth

Lisa Jennison, University of Hull

Daniel Kelly, Cardiff University

Fiona Timmins, Trinity College Dublin

Roger Watson, University of Hull

INTRODUCTION

Success is not final, failure is not fatal: it is the courage to continue that counts.

Winston Churchill

In the week where we finally delivered this manuscript to our publishers, the unveiling of a statue of suffragist Millicent Fawcett, an important figure in the votes for women campaign, had just taken place in Parliament Square. She was sculpted holding a banner with the words, 'Courage speaks to courage everywhere'.[1]

Delivering good healthcare demands both rational and emotional work, and it is this emotional work that requires courage of those involved. Courage is both contextual and a highly personal phenomenon. For example, at the point of submission of this book, one of the authors does not know how soon it will be before his own mother passes away, or whether an operation to clear bleeding in one of his eyes will allow restoration of sight ever again.

The idea for this book came about after the authors had written a blogpost, asking the question, '*Are we contributing to a culture of fear?*' Recognising that what gets talked about gets attention, the authors wanted to get people to think about how every day, across the work of those in health and social care, everyone – be they leaders, politicians, staff, patients or 'service users' – is pursuing difficult 'life' and 'work' narratives that require them to draw on their emotional and moral courage. The junior doctor in the emergency department who has to tell a relative that the urgent scan shows there is widespread cancer; the medical secretary who takes the call from the husband and tells them their wife has committed suicide following their diagnosis; the patient who is told they have a degenerative illness which will threaten their whole identity and have profound impact on their role as the main earner in the family; the middle manager who has to tell the surgeon she cannot operate as there are no beds.

All of these situations require courage and *people to be supported* in doing this work. Yet, we hear people say that staff need to have courage to speak up when they have concerns or admit they have made a mistake. Patients talk of the fear of making a complaint in case of eliciting a punitive response. We believe that this should not require courage and if it does, it tells us that the culture and relationships in which this courage is required are dysfunctional and need attention. It is striking that, in the limited literature which exists on courage, the emphasis has been on the individual rather than the wider environment.

---

[1] See: www.theguardian.com/politics/2018/apr/25/misgivings-over-new-statue-and-old-portrait-of-millicent-fawcett

We know that it is in this second area that courage gets the most attention.

The main observation is that the call for courage can have both negative and positive outcomes. It can be beneficial for enabling therapeutic relationships and diverse aspects such as wellbeing and innovation, but it can be a negative experience even if there are benefits 'against the odds' such as in whistleblowing.

We wanted to explore with the reader the everyday courage in the work of healthcare so that it gets recognised, valued and nurtured, and to look at how the current experience of overcoming fear to question and challenge the 'system' can be changed to a more positive one where questioning and pointing out risks is 'just the way things get done around here.

We have divided the book into separate chapters but want to emphasise that these issues are all connected and it is only by looking at things in their entirety that we understand the true complexity of why healthcare requires the courage of all who are involved in it.

We have tried to write in a way to get you to think about the subject but also the role that you do and could play in creating the conditions for courage when needed to flourish, whilst removing the need for it when it should not be required.

In the end, all of us contribute to the circumstances we encounter, and it is in recognising that, that we can draw on our power and influence to make a positive difference together.

About this book

This book looks at courage in healthcare from various points of view of the people involved, ranging from politicians to professionals, manager or leader, to patient or service user. The book is not intended to be an all-inclusive, complete analysis of courage, but is intended as a launchpad for us all to respond to the sensitive issues which courage often ensnares. We have deliberately tried to emphasise that these issues do not belong to 'silos' of particular people, but cut through a range of different experiences. In our attempt to combine the research in this area with the everyday practices and experiences of healthcare, there are aspects of this book you might find highly technocratic, but others which you find highly personal too.

Chapter 1 – What is courage?

As individuals, 'courage' as a cognitive and behavioural characteristic involves both a response from the mind and body, and the cognitive processes of decision making in the face of risk and uncertainty whilst perceiving fear. Courage in individuals can contribute to courage in organisations, but the context of this is all-important. Courage notably can be intimately linked with other traits such as compassion or resilience. This chapter will look at the neurocognitive processes of courage, but will also look at how courage, whilst called for in NHS policy,[2] can be linked all the way back to the philosophies of Plato and Aristotle. But a major gap in our understanding is how whole systems determine the manifestations of individual courage, and this gap will unfortunately manifest itself throughout the book.

Chapter 2 – Courage to care

Courage to care and courage in being a carer are quite profoundly different things. This chapter is about the 'courage to care'. Health and social care professionals are subject to constraints in time and finances, which may compromise their ability to care, and these can also be pertinent for unpaid family carers.

To care for another requires you to become emotionally involved. Being emotionally involved can mean you are vulnerable and get hurt and this is why it takes courage to care. However, if you believe that a central tenet of care is not just what you *do to* someone but caring *about* them as a fellow human being, it is impossible not to get involved.

Chapter 3 – Courage to lead

Courage is also critical to people who run the NHS and social services. Lessons can be drawn from the leadership styles of people who have brought about and exhibited great courage, bringing widespread change, such as Gandhi or Martin Luther King. But courage to lead doesn't have to be of the charismatic variety, but could simply be transformative or technocratic in approach in achieving healthcare targets. It could be possible to 'measure' courage one day, to solidify it as a desirable characteristic.

By the nature of the work, healthcare requires difficult decisions to be made. Stepping forward to lead in any scenario, whether as the domestic on the ward to offer a suggestion on how to do something different, or the decision of a politician to invest in some services at the expense of others, can be difficult. When these decisions are filled with difficult emotions such as fear of getting it wrong, distress at the impact it will have, or upset, leading requires courage.

Chapter 4 – Courage to live and die

Courage can be extremely personal too. Courage historically has been couched in the language of adversarial combat, and this runs in parallel with media messaging about conditions such as cancer or dementia. This chapter will consider whether it

---

[2]See *Compassion in Practice: Nursing, Midwifery and Care Staff – Our Vision and Strategy*, 2012, Department of Health

is appropriate to consider cancer or dementia as a 'fight' – in that there are some cancers, for example, where complete remission is a possibility. The alternative will be considered where rehabilitation with a long-term condition is positively promoted. The chapter will conclude with personal reflections on coping with potential death. While anything can happen to anyone at any time, the preparation for death is important, for example, in palliative approaches; and has implications for individual reactions to life-changing illnesses and the lives of close carers.

Chapter 5 – Courage to challenge

The CIPD defines someone as having 'the courage to challenge' as someone who 'shows courage and confidence to speak up skilfully, challenging others even when confronted with resistance or unfamiliar circumstances'.[3] This chapter has as its focus an extreme form of such a challenge – colloquially called 'whistleblowing'. The term 'blow the whistle' has long been felt to be a strong phraseology for the courage to speak up against negative work cultures where things have gone wrong. Problems have still remained pursuant to the Public Interest Disclosure Act (1998) which is supposed to protect public sector employees. And yet speaking up courageously is often needed to promote patient safety, a key duty of all registrants in healthcare. This chapter will describe the individual experiences of people who have spoken out against the system, including misdiagnosis of important conditions, criticising poor clinical care and speaking out against child abuse. A more helpful way of framing these sensitive issues might therefore be a 'courage to challenge', in a way that promotes teamwork and conflict resolution. Unfortunately, too often people who speak out find themselves emotionally and intellectually 'burnt out', and the chapter will consider the pivotal need to protect staff wellbeing too. The chapter will consider why the narrative is framed so much in an adversarial way, and how possible ways forward could mean that it is easier to have courage to speak out in future.

Chapter 6 – Courage to flourish

The chapter will consider how a more substantial re-thinking about healthcare systems might be needed, such as a less retributive approach to healthcare regulation and a more inclusive way of organising and providing healthcare that opens it up to more diverse views on what is happening and why, in order to promote organisational development and learning. We will try to bring together some of the themes which have emerged in our discussion of courage in this book. Fundamental to thinking about how courage can 'flourish' is the answer to the question:

---

[3]See: www.cipd.co.uk/Images/Courage-to-Challenge_tcm18-9692.pdf

Under what professional, personal and environmental conditions should someone need to show courage and when does the need for courage suggest there is a problem?

A final note

Writing this book has not been without its own challenges. For one of the authors trying to care for his mother as her needs accumulate, whilst juggling personal physical health issues, has required huge courage to keep going. Finding a way to write together from very different backgrounds and experiences and accepting we disagree about different aspects of the work have created the courage to be honest with each other about our different interpretations of events. We have also negotiated the balance of the academic literature on this subject with the day-to-day reality of working in the NHS.

We hope that you find some of the topics which we discuss interesting and relevant to your views, research or form of practice, and will motivate you to think about possible avenues for further exploration in this important area.

1

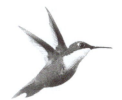

WHAT IS COURAGE?

SHIBLEY RAHMAN

I learned that courage was not the absence of fear, but the triumph over it. The brave man is not he who does not feel afraid, but he who conquers that fear.

Nelson Mandela

Introduction

This chapter lays the foundations for the 'arena' of courage, but, as we will see in the coming chapters, courage is in fact a very fertile phenomenon for all involved in healthcare systems, and there are in fact many wider issues to discuss. Many of them do not, in fact, lend themselves easily to traditional academic analysis, but require an evolving, organic narrative to develop of its own accord.

It is essential that the healthcare sector develops leaders with strong ethical values, who are willing to live these values with integrity and courage, even when doing so risks their position in the hierarchy of the organisation (Murray, 2010). There are millions of examples of courage in healthcare, all very different. At the time of preparation of this manuscript, the High Court had just ruled that doctors could withdraw life support from a sick baby with a rare genetic condition against his parents' wishes. Specialists at Great Ormond Street Hospital said eight-month-old Charlie Gard had irreversible brain damage and should be given palliative care. His parents, from London, had wanted to take him to the US for a treatment trial. 'Hope' is that much-valued scarce resource in clinical care. The parents unsurprisingly said they were 'devastated' by the Court's decision but intended to appeal. In the summary provided contemporaneously, to assist understanding of the Court's decision handed down on Tuesday 11 April 2017, the Judge had written in conclusion:

> I want to thank the team of experts and carers at GOSH, and others who cannot be named, for the extraordinary care that they have provided to this family. Most importantly of all, I want to thank Charlie's parents for their brave and dignified campaign on his behalf, but more than anything to pay tribute to their absolute dedication to their wonderful boy, from the day that he was born. (Judiciary of England and Wales, 2017)

At approximately the same time, the family of Keith Palmer, the police officer stabbed to death by a terrorist as he guarded the Palace of Westminster, paid tribute to a 'wonderful dad and husband' who was 'dedicated to his job, brave and courageous'.

Examples of actual courageous individuals are indeed far too numerous to mention, but some are provided in Box 1.1.

Box 1.1:   Courageous figures in history

Socrates (469 BC–399 BC)

A Greek philosopher, Socrates was willing to die for his beliefs. Arrested for his philosophic teachings, Socrates was willing to accept death rather than change his opinions and beliefs. It is said he calmly accepted his fate.

Emmeline Pankhurst (1858–1928)

Pankhurst was a militant campaigner for women's right to vote, who along with many other suffragettes was imprisoned because of her protesting. Her philosophy was that the need to extend voting rights to women was so urgent that breaking the law in order to draw attention to the cause was completely justified. She was imprisoned several times, but saw her goals realised when women were allowed to vote for the first time in 1918.

Dietrich Bonhoeffer (1906–1945)

This German Lutheran pastor was consistently outspoken in his criticism of Nazism in Germany. Preferring to stay in the country of his birth, he was eventually arrested and executed in Flossian concentration camp.

Nelson Mandela (1918–2013)

Nelson Mandela had the courage to fight against the unjust system of apartheid. For his political activities, he was sentenced to 20 years in prison, but he was released to lead a free South Africa.

Malala Yousafzai (1997–)

Malala is a Pakistani activist for female education and the youngest ever Nobel Prize laureate. She is known for human rights advocacy, especially the education of women in her native Swat Valley in Khyber Pakhtunkhwa, northwest Pakistan, where the local Taliban had at times banned girls from attending school. Her advocacy has since grown into an international movement.

Why is 'courage' important?

The phenomenon of 'having courage' is a universal lived experience of health that is significant to quality of life (Bournes, 2002).

> Having courage is a human experience intertwined with all life events – embracing meaning and values, desires and dreams, relationships and plans, concerns and fears. It is an experience that everyone can describe in some way in relation to their own lives. It is a particularly vivid experience for persons who have had to find ways to move on with their lives amid the challenges inherent with learning to live with a spinal cord injury. (2002: 220)

A possible reason why courage has not received more attention and formal inquiry thus far may be attributed to difficulties in establishing a clear and concise definition. One reason Woodard and Pury (2007) offer in explaining the lack of research is the difficulty in establishing a clear and concise definition of the multidimensional construct. The question of interest is what do these examples of 'courage' have in common? If we wish to apply learning about courage to individuals and organisations in healthcare, where do we start? Stories of courage or the lack of it have long fascinated listeners. Shakespeare's *Hamlet*, a tragedy that is just as relevant today, tells of Hamlet's struggle to muster enough courage to confront the murderer of his father.

The precise definition of courage may not be settled yet. But courage is very relevant to how staff, including experienced professionals and practitioners, have to operate, perhaps in understaffed conditions with 'efficiency savings'. There is, for example, an intense fear that you might be deemed 'underperforming' if you cannot work at a pace and still maintain patient safety. The focus of any health and social care service, now and into the future, should be people delivering safe, quality care to people; care that covers not just diagnosis and treatment, but the whole experience that patients and their carers have of the service.

Some organisations have been shown to be poor employers with a culture of bullying and fear and the use of suspensions and financial settlements bound to gagging clauses to remove whistleblowers; furthermore, issues of gender and ethnic discrimination do not get fully resolved (Easmon, 2014). In one survey of over 624,000 staff, 93% indicated that they knew how to report concerns; however, only 57% expressed the view that they were confident that their concerns would be addressed (NHS, 2014). The solution therefore is to ensure that the focus should be on the culture within an organisation to ameliorate the need for disaffected staff to take the courageous step of reporting outside to effect action and bring to a close the offending practice or practices. When health service managers are faced with reports of failure and particularly issues that raise concerns about patient safety, they will demonstrate a human response.

Surely, then, a 'courage to challenge' is important? That will be the focus of Chapter 5.

What seems to be unknown at this time are the 'human factors' involved in the behaviours of healthcare managers who distance themselves from staff who raise concerns about patient safety (Cleary and Doyle, 2015). This is of particular relevance to clinical managers who are part of healthcare administration, managing clinicians who are the greatest number of health staff. Clinical managers are working at different levels in healthcare organisations: ward, middle and strategic management. They have ethical responsibilities to the healthcare organisation, to patients cared for in this organisation and to the clinical staff employed by this organisation. Clinical managers play a role in clarifying organisations' mission, vision and values to their staff (Aitamaa et al., 2016).

'Human factors' are very relevant to courage, and are much discussed at various points in this book.

What is 'courage'?

You will get your 'own feel' for what courage is and is not, as you progress through this book, perhaps relating to your own personal experiences.

In an article by Kathleen K. Reardon in *Harvard Business Review* (2007: 60), a 'courage calculation' is even described thus:

> Learning to take an intelligent gamble requires an understanding of what I call the 'courage calculation': a method of making success more likely while avoiding rash, unproductive, or irrational behaviour. Six discrete processes make up the courage calculation: setting primary and secondary goals; determining the importance of achieving them; tipping the power balance in your favor; weighing risks against benefits; selecting the proper time for action; and developing contingency plans.

Courage has been described as the will to accomplish a goal in the face of opposition or risk (Peterson and Seligman, 2004). Courage comes from feeling very deeply about important values and working to achieve goals that are consistent with those values. Clinicians and practitioners often find themselves in situations where they are morally obligated to take risks, within a certain range of reasonableness, in order to secure the rights and welfare of their patients.

In his third 2014 BBC Reith Lecture, entitled 'the problem of hubris', Boston surgeon Atul Gawande lamented what he saw as the over-medicalising of patients in their final days and moments: 'Doctors ... can deny people these moments, relegating them to the care of strangers alone in an intensive care unit' and 'the way we can forget this out of obtuseness and neglect, is I think cause for our shame' (cited in Iles, 2016: 105).

Healthcare systems are in a perpetual state of flux and change (Naylor and Naylor, 2012). Driving clinical practice innovation requires not only leadership at a senior level but the directing of staff towards shared values and a vision for improving patient care (Davidson et al., 2013). Leaders generate morally courageous behaviour by fostering relational, contextual and motivational support in followers. The interpersonal trust created through relational support facilitates moral courage by mitigating the inherent risk involved in balancing stakeholder interest while support, which creates a sense of mission and purpose, promotes courageous action (Hernandez, 2008). Innovation itself requires a willingness to take risks and an ability to be courageous in coping with failure. A country's football manager might go on to lead his team successfully even if he has himself missed a crucial penalty as a footballer many years previously. Ethics is the study of standards of conduct and moral judgements as well as the study of what is considered to be right or acceptable behaviour and what is considered wrong (Jenson, 1997), and is clearly relevant to the practice of 'courage' in healthcare settings.

In trying to identify what is 'courageous', one can observe that 'you recognise it when you see it'. Individuals who are courageous, regardless of setting, tend to be so despite huge risk to themselves, for a very serious cause. But does character reflect character either in business or healthcare? The study of character in courage in modern organisational units is relatively scant (Sarros et al., 2006). Character has been defined as 'doing the right thing despite outside pressure to the contrary' (Likona, 1991). To act with character, arguably, is to exhibit virtue. Tjeltveit (2003: 400) comments: 'character and virtue have to do with the ethical qualities of persons, with what we view as good, or excellent, or praiseworthy about them'.

Virtues are central to character, both personally and professionally; virtues and other moral traits are widely regarded by the general public as important aspects of personality, even though personality researchers have yet to research their interrelationship fully. A recent philosophical account contends that virtues 'come closer to defining who the person is than any other category of qualities' (Zagzebski, 1996: 135). Indeed, education philosopher Parker Palmer (1990) illustrates this phenomenon by using the example of Americans' reaction to Rosa Parks. In 1955, Rosa Parks, a highly respected civil rights activist, defied the law by refusing to give up her seat to a white man aboard a city bus in Montgomery, Alabama. Parks' arrest sparked major demonstrations that subsequently led to important advances in US civil rights legislation. Palmer made it clear that if Rosa Parks' story is to support our own courage to stand up for what we care most about,

> We must see her as the ordinary person she is. That will be difficult to do because we have made her into superwoman – and we have done it to protect ourselves. If we can keep Rosa Parks in a museum as an untouchable icon of truth, we will remain untouchable as well: we can put her up on a pedestal and praise her, world without end, never finding ourselves challenged by her life. (1990: 35)

Courage, conviction and healthcare often go together.

Daring to care requires courage – the courage to speak out and to act. Courage transforms convictions and compassion into action (Adler and Hansen, 2012). There is, therefore, a broad consensus on a definition of courage:

> Courage is the ability to face the fear, acknowledge it, and live through it. Courage is a human trait or virtue that is, in a broad sense, the ability of an individual or group to overcome actual or perceived threat or loss in order to achieve another outcome. (Crigger and Godfrey, 2011: 13)

Rachman (1984), in trying to understand why some people respond to fear in a manner that might be conducive to courageous behaviour, studied paratroopers. His assessment of subjective fear and the corresponding physiological markers revealed that paratroopers reported a moderate amount of fear at the beginning of their programme, but this fear subsided within their initial five jumps. Furthermore, it was found that the execution of a jump despite the presence of fear (i.e. courage) resulted in a reduction of fear. Rachman (1984) suggested that courage was related to resilience in the face of threat or danger, and perseverance or the capacity to act despite stress and fear. Rachman concludes by suggesting that training or exposure to the fearful situation may move the person along on a type of continuum, from courage to fearlessness. There is such a notion, according to the Greeks – and most of us would agree – as excessive fearlessness. A person who exudes too much confidence when he or she should be fearful is considered rash.

Courage has been defined by Rachman (1984, 2004) as a 'behavioural approach in spite of the experience of fear'. Rachman's (1984, 2004) conceptualisation of courage as approach behaviour in combination with fear also seems relevant to clinical psychology, and in particular to the domain of fear, anxiety and their disorders. When facing threat, those who engage in courageous behaviour by exposing themselves to the feared stimulus or situation, are less likely to develop serious anxiety problems (Muris, 2009). In contrast, those who display a tendency to avoid and act cowardly will show a continuation and exacerbation of their fears (Mowrer, 1960).

Norton and Weiss (2009) conducted a study to assess courage, defined as a behavioural approach despite the experience of fear, in an effort to better understand its relationship with anxiety, fear and the behavioural approach. This study advanced knowledge about the relationship between courage and fear. Future studies can explore the extent to which (*a*) courage mediates the willingness to engage in therapeutic exposure in treatment, and (*b*) whether courage can be augmented in treatment prior to implementing exposure therapy.

On the basis of six qualitative studies with individuals aged 14 to 94 years experiencing various threats to their wellbeing, Finfgeld (1999: 803) published a meta-interpretation to synthesise an emergent theory of courage:

> Courageous behaviour is characterized by efforts to be productive, make contributions, and help others and results in a sense of personal integrity and thriving. Courage is promoted and sustained by several interrelated intrapersonal and interpersonal forces as well as the reflective awareness that one has developed a courageous persona.

Shelp described courage as 'the disposition to voluntarily act, perhaps fearfully, in a dangerous circumstance, where the relevant risks are reasonably appraised, in an effort to obtain or preserve some perceived good for oneself or others' (1984: 345). Shelp (1984) proposed four components of courage: (1) free choice to accept or not accept the consequences of acting, (2) risk or danger, (3) a worthy end, and (4) uncertainty of outcome. He indicated that fear may or may not be present in the courageous act.

The idea that courage is not the preserve of the exceptional few, and that we can all look for acts of courage in our lives, opens the way to a new appreciation of the old understanding of courage. Courage has historically been regarded as a great virtue because it helps people to face their intrapersonal and interpersonal challenges. Virtue ethics, in general, has concentrated on what is required to produce a good person with good character, implying that right action will somehow flow from the right set of moral dispositions. Enlightenment moral theorists set questions of character aside, contending that what really mattered was either the production of the best overall consequences (utilitarianism) or the agent's intent to do the right thing solely because it was one's duty (Kantianism).

From a humanistic point of view, clinicians require virtue of courage not only to be a good human but also to provide an acceptable care level for their patient, the family and society. Meanwhile, for professional growth in nursing, professional values such as courage need to be developed to perform functions and decisions properly and to avoid chaos and damage (Sadooghiasl et al., 2016). Anticipated emotions – what we expect to feel in a future situation – may also be influential in this type of decision making (e.g. Perugini and Bagozzi, 2004).

Overlap between courage and other kinds of behaviours

Caring with courage often involves actions that go beyond the call of duty, actions that can properly be called heroic. Take, for example, those healthcare volunteers working to combat the highly infectious and potent *Ebola* virus. Courage clearly overlaps with other closely related behaviours. For example:

> Heroism can be viewed as a highly moral behaviour that has been explained as a form of sensation-seeking, altruism, citizenship and bravery and as a desirable but sometimes non-adaptive response in Darwinian terms. All these behaviours seem to involve some sort of emotional trigger and usually a rapid response. (Harvey et al., 2000: 313)

One form of heroism is 'courageous resistance', defined as a voluntary selfless behaviour in which there is significantly high risk or cost to the individual and possibly their family and associates; not all altruistic people will exhibit this, and those who do are not always courageous (Shepela, 1999). The idea of 'courageous resistance' can be extended to behaviours such as whistleblowing (Glazer and Glazer, 1999). A physical symbol of this was seen in a stark example on 5 June 1989. One day after the Chinese government's violent crackdown on the Tiananmen protests, a man placed himself directly in the path of a column of tanks that were approaching the Square. He acted alone, holding nothing but one shopping bag in each hand.

But, crucially, one has to consider whether these other behaviours or attributes are an artefact of a system in which a person operates with courage. Does a person who is courageous have to be so 'heroic' because he or she is operating in such a 'hostile environment'?

A historical perspective

Aquinas described courage as a 'general virtue' (Dierksmeier and Celano, 2012), whilst Samuel Johnson said that 'courage is reckoned the greatest of all virtues; because unless a man has that virtue he has no security for preserving any other' (Miller, 2000: 5). Scholars have debated the various meanings of 'courage' over the centuries.

Ancient Greek philosophers frequently used the term in reference to character on the battlefield. Plato and Aristotle discussed courage as a trait set aside for situations where individuals feared death. Aristotle in his *Nicomachean Ethics* is perhaps the best-known advocate that the proper sphere of courage is solely the battlefield. There has, of course, been an enduring imagery of healthcare as a 'fight' or 'battle', so it is perhaps not surprising to see courage appear in this context: 'A culture of individual heroism and "tough-mindedness" has defined western medicine for nearly 400 years, and this can be characterised as a culture with a "love of war", where confrontation, anger and bullying are endemic' (Bleakley et al., 2014: 22).

Courage is recognised as a valuable human character trait and its central place in ethics and moral life can be traced at least back to Aristotle (384–322 BC) (Lindh et al., 2010). The virtues and vices according to Aristotle are summarised by Ladikos (2004). In Aristotle's view the moral *virtues*, on the one side, include: courage, temperance, self-discipline, moderation, modesty, humility, generosity, friendliness, truthfulness, honesty, justice. The moral *vices*, on the other side, include: cowardice, self-indulgence, recklessness, wastefulness, greed, vanity, untruthfulness, dishonesty, injustice. Acts of virtue bring honour to an individual, whilst acts of vice bring dishonour to an individual. Aristotelian military courage (*andreia*) is concerned with the passions of fear (*phobos*) and confidence (*tharsos*). It is thus exhibited in the face of what is fearful and dangerous. Ladikos (2004) also helpfully considers the derivation of courage in Ancient Greek. The Greek word for courage is '*andreia*' which literally means manly courage or bravery; moreover, it refers to the state or quality of mind or spirit that enables one to face danger, fear or vicissitudes with self-possession and resolution. It is a mental or moral strength to face danger with fear and reflects the quality of mind or spirit that enables one to face difficulty, danger, pain and any adverse circumstances.

It is argued that Aristotle finds echoes in approaches in modern management. For example, Kurzynski (2012) argues that a careful reading of Peter Drucker's works reveals that there is much in his management philosophy that is analogous with Aristotle's moral philosophy as delineated in the *Nicomachean Ethics*, and to some degree with his political philosophy as delineated in *The Politics*. For example, Drucker aligned with professional responsibility the duty to act with integrity, exercise sound judgement and courage, and '[a]bove all, not knowingly to do harm' (Drucker, 1973: 268–269).

Plato's most famous work, many might agree, is *The Republic*. Though generally regarded as a Utopian presentation of justice, it actually discusses the four cardinal virtues – justice, wisdom, moderation and courage – and other topics, including friendship, 'the good' for the individual and the city-state (*polis*) (Alvey, 2011). The term 'cardinal' comes from the Latin cardo (hinge); the cardinal virtues are so called because they are regarded as the basic virtues required for a virtuous life. Plato's earliest treatment of the theme of courage is in the dialogue *Laches* (Plato, 1973). Socrates is one of many who sought to understand this noble quality, as illustrated in his question to Laches: 'Suppose we set about determining the nature of courage and in the second place, proceed to inquire how the young men may attain this quality by the help of study and pursuits. Tell me, if you can, what is courage', implored Socrates (Plato, 1973).

The question of 'what is courage?' has always garnered significant interest and debate, from the work of Plato, and without necessarily providing an agreed consensus definition. What is agreed is that there are many different types of courage and many different situations that call for courage. There, his spokesperson, Socrates, is faced with the title character, a general who is quite convinced that he is courageous when others can easily see that his behaviour is dangerously rash. If courage is what Laches thinks it is, it certainly does not seem worth recommending.

As we see in Plato's *Laches* dialogue, Socrates offered an incredibly broad definition of courage that accounted for every single instance in which courageous action might be possible. He wanted to take into account and consider how courage related to everyday common activities such as facing individual sicknesses, poverty, pains and fears. Socrates even believed that animals possessed a certain degree of courage. Plato was always aware that people who thought they were acting courageously could be prone to producing negative outcomes (Raffel, 2011). Raffel finds that: 'Arguably, *The Republic* has a less arbitrary way of defending the need for courage while resisting negatives associated with it' (2011: 91).

One other scholarly description, that of the Roman statesman Cicero (as summarised by Houser, 2002), may be the view of courage that best transcends time. Houser noted that Cicero saw courage as:

> (1) magnificence, the planning and execution of great and expansive projects by putting forth ample and splendid effort of mind; (2) confidence, that through which, on great and honorable projects, the mind self-confidently collects itself with sure hope; (3) patience, the voluntary and lengthy endurance of arduous and difficult things, whether the case be honorable or useful; and (4) perseverance, ongoing persistence in a well-considered plan. (2002: 305)

A neurocognitive perspective

How the mind and brain 'process' courage gives us clues about its relevance. The timescale of the 'courageous response' is important, and the fact that the construct is multifaceted will have differing neural substrates.

Hawkins and Morse (2014: 267) observe that:

> Courage can also be reflexive and instantaneous, or more slowly reflective as a result of a premeditated difficult decision and subsequent action. It follows that if courage is an overwhelming reflexive response—one that is stronger than fear in or for one's self, one that is almost an impulsive sense of duty—then courage is a different concept from care and is manifested as stronger than a caring action.

But how much courage is reflexive or reactionary to events or people, rather than anticipatory, is an important issue in neurocognition.

Courageous actions exhibit thoughtful deliberation, although there might be an impulsive, retributive component. On the other hand, courageous behaviours are usually characterised by performance of voluntary actions in a response to underlying fear. Experimentally using functional neuroimaging, by distinguishing defined actions of either overcoming fear or succumbing to it in an acute controllable fearful situation, one can possibly identify underlying neural substrates of courage (e.g. Nili et al., 2010). There is converging evidence that many people overestimate how frightened they will be when faced with a fear-provoking situation. This over prediction of fear is commonly seen in people who are troubled by excessive fear (e.g. people who are prone to panic or claustrophobia), but is not confined to them (Rachman, 1994).

To initiate a courageous response, there needs to be a trigger, and the level of threat proposed by this trigger needs to be assessed, perhaps by comparison to similar triggers in the past. The accuracy of this assessment is likely to be affected by your general state of motivation and arousal. Hannah et al. (2007) have proposed a theory explaining how the individual may experience courage on a subjective level and how these experiences may lead to the development of what they call 'a courageous mind-set' (2007: 129). In the model of Hannah and colleagues, factors such as the perception of risk are impacted by external constructs such as social forces (e.g. normative influences) and positive states (such as hope, efficacy or the experience of positive emotions), as well as more internal characteristics such as positive traits (e.g. openness to experience and conscientiousness) and values and beliefs (e.g. loyalty, honour). These authors posit that these influences have a collective effect on how risk is perceived, how fear is experienced and whether courageous behaviours are exhibited.

The relationship between courage and confidence is indeed an interesting one. In a novel experiment, McMillan and Rachman (1988) investigated whether trainees of a parachute jump could be reliably grouped into clusters of 'courageous' and 'fearless' jumpers. The results of their analysis are fascinating, with distinctions drawn between 'fearless' and 'courageous' performances. Courageous individuals had relatively modest expectations about jumping and became, by and large, more positive following their first aeroplane jump. The profile of 'fearless' individuals contrasted markedly. About one-quarter of the sample fell into this category which represented recruits who were highly confident before jumping and expected relatively low levels of fear and danger. The neural substrates underlying these phenomena have yet to be elucidated.

Courageous action involves voluntarily pursuing a socially worthy goal despite the accompanying risk and the fear produced by a challenging event. At present, little research exists on the factors that describe the antecedents, enablers and processes of courageous actions (Schilpzand et al., 2014). Woodard (2004) examined the role that courage plays in the construct of hardiness as a mediator between hardiness and physical health. 'Hardiness' is a personality style or pattern associated with performance under stress (Kobasa, 1979). Rate's conception of courage, which involves both personal risks and noble goals, provides a framework for understanding different types of courage in terms of risk–goal pairs (Rate, 2010; Rate et al., 2007). But even then, this approach is individualistic, and speaks little to the wider environment in which a person is functioning.

Rate and colleagues, through qualitative research, offer this detailed definition:

a. a willful, intentional act,
b. executed after mindful deliberation,
c. involving objective substantial risk to the actor,
d. primarily motivated to bring about a noble good or worthy end
e. despite perhaps the presence of the emotion of fear. (2007: 95)

A recent study investigates the relationship between courage, personality traits and coping strategies, hypothesising that courage could mediate between personality and coping (Magnano et al., 2017). The participants were 500 Italian adults, aged 18 to 60, paired for gender. The results showed that courage can be considered a mediator between personality and coping, affecting the use of self-directed strategies. Interpersonal factors, such as role models, also help to promote and maintain courage. Courageous individuals model exemplary behaviour that they have observed throughout their lives, in particular commendable conduct that has been exhibited by immediate and extended family members (reviewed in Finfgeld, 1999).

It is possible to obtain an impression of the neural substrates of cognition relevant to courage from the existing literature. Organisational dysfunction has numerous outcomes, from the lack of an appropriate fit between the organisation and its environment, through the inappropriate composition of task-based management teams, to the incompatible predispositions and behavioural styles of individual managers. Theories of managerial behaviour and, in particular, prescriptions that derive from them, require a cognitive understanding of the nature of decision making (Foxall, 2014).

The *somatic marker hypothesis* proposes that decision making is a process that depends on emotion. Studies have shown that damage of the ventromedial prefrontal cortex precludes the ability to use somatic (emotional) signals that are necessary for guiding decisions in an advantageous direction (Bechara et al., 1999). Decades of animal and human research have shown that the amygdala is involved in conditioned and unconditioned responses to stimuli. It is believed that the amygdala is involved in coupling a stimulus which evokes an emotional response (i.e. a primary inducer, such as a snake) with its affective value. The evidence for this comes not only from fear conditioning work, but also from the classic work of Klüver and Bucy (1939) who showed that monkeys with mesial temporal lesions that included the amygdala have an increased tendency to approach emotionally salient stimuli, such as snakes (Gupta et al., 2011).

Risk and individual differences

To the ethologist, the terms fear and anxiety are survival responses and reflect broad categories, each having their own behavioural and contextual profile (Mobbs and Kim, 2015). According to the risk allocation hypothesis, animals allocate most of their defensive resources to situations of high predator threat (Lima and Bednekoff, 1999). In the last few years, neuroscientists have begun to identify associations between individual differences in decision making and features of neuroanatomy and neurophysiology. Different tendencies in decision making, such as tolerance for risk, delay or effort, have been linked to various neurobiological measures, such as morphometry, structural connectivity, functional connectivity or the function of neurotransmitter systems (Kable and Levy, 2015).

Age differences in decision quality and risk aversion are likely to have different psychological roots. The ability to identify the option with the higher expected value requires, by definition, the ability to integrate risk and reward information and might therefore rest on fluid abilities, which decline in older age; the degree of risk aversion, by contrast, seems to be shaped more by emotional than by cognitive factors (Pachur et al., 2017). Decision making and individual mood have a complex interrelationship. Optimism and pessimism – expecting a positive or negative future – are distinct modes of thinking that are best conceptualised not rigidly and dichotomously but rather as a continuum with many degrees of optimism and pessimism. A person can be optimistic in regard to a specific area of life (e.g. expecting his/her marriage/relationship to succeed) but pessimistic regarding other aspects (e.g. expecting financial difficulties ahead) (Hecht, 2013).

The perception and accurate assessment of risk in future events is important for both patients and clinicians. Consider, for example, risk stratification for open heart surgery. If you are awaiting open heart surgery, you might use the information in working out whether you are 'courageous' enough to have open heart surgery. On the other hand, for the clinical provider, the information could be used for prioritising selection from waiting lists, advising referring doctors and patients of the expected outcome of different treatment options, or analysing resource use. Decision making relating to future events is dependent on neural processes. Intertemporal decision making refers to the process of choosing between rewards that differ in the amount and time to delivery. It is the basis for long-term planning of personal matters such as financial issues and health-related behaviours (Hu et al., 2017). During intertemporal decision making, people frequently give preference to smaller immediate rewards rather than (even greater) future rewards. This tendency to devalue future rewards as opposed to immediate rewards is termed delay discounting (Ainslie, 1975).

During the process of collaborative decision making, humans may influence and bias each other's decision making. When examining the decision-making processes during 'fiascos', Janis described the process of *groupthink* that he felt led to poor decision making (Janis, 1982). Janis defined groupthink as 'a mode of thinking people engage in when they are deeply involved in a cohesive in-group, when the members striving for unanimity override their motivation to realistically appraise alternative courses of action' (Kaba et al., 2016). Peer effects have also been shown to affect individual choice under risk. Yechiam and colleagues (2008) let subjects make binary choices under risk on a computer while looking at a real-time broadcast from another subject's choice screen, thus exposing subjects to each other's choices and outcomes. The authors reported that mutual observation in pairs led to higher risk-taking, but this effect was not observed when only one of the subjects in the pair observed the other.

We will resume the discussion of risks, in particular 'calculated risks', in Chapter 6 in discussing innovation.

The '6Cs'

The 6Cs, which underpin the 'Compassion in Practice' strategy[1], were developed in England as a way of articulating the values which need to underpin the culture and practice of organisations delivering care and support. These are immediately identifiable as values which underpin quality social care provision too. As integration between health and social care continues and increases, it is helpful to focus on common values expressed in ways which increase consistency within all aspects of work, workforce, leadership and organisations. The 6Cs were launched in December 2012. In *Compassion in Practice* the 6Cs are defined as shown in Box 1.2.

Box 1.2:   The 6Cs

Care: is our core business and that of our organisations, and the care we deliver helps the individual person and improves the health of the whole community. Caring defines us and our work. People receiving care expect it to be right for them, consistently, throughout every stage of their life.

Compassion: is how care is given through relationships based on empathy, respect and dignity – it can also be described as intelligent kindness, and is central to how people perceive their care.

Competence: means all those in caring roles must have the ability to understand an individual's health and social needs and the expertise, clinical and technical knowledge to deliver effective care and treatments based on research and evidence.

Communication: is central to successful caring relationships and to effective team working. Listening is as important as what we say and do and essential for 'no decision about me without me'. Communication is the key to a good workplace with benefits for those in our care and staff alike.

Courage: enables us to do the right thing for the people we care for, to speak up when we have concerns and to have the personal strength and vision to innovate and to embrace new ways of working.

Commitment: to our patients and populations is a cornerstone of what we do. We need to build on our commitment to improve the care and experience of our patients, to take action to make this vision and strategy a reality for all and meet the health, care and support challenges ahead.

Source: NHS Commissioning Board/Department of Health (2012) *Compassion in Practice: Nursing, Midwifery and Care Staff – Our Vision and Strategy*. Available at: www.england.nhs.uk/wp-content/uploads/2012/12/compassion-in-practice.pdf

---

[1]See: https://www.england.nhs.uk/wp-content/uploads/2012/12/compassion-in-practice.pdf

Examples given by NHS England (2013) include: courage to speak up, courage to raise concerns, courage in not being afraid to explore difficult scenarios, courage from the nursing team to trial a system that their colleagues are not using, and courage to involve nurses working in an autonomous way.

It is interesting to observe the centrality of dignity. As David Albert Jones observes (Jones, 2015: 90):

> In relation to healthcare both these elements of observing people's dignity will be important, but before looking at respect and obedience in this context, it is useful to draw attention to another distinction Thomas makes, between what he calls special virtue (virtus specialis) and general virtue (virtus generalis). This is best illustrated by an example. Courage is a virtue of our assertive emotions that enables us to act well in fearful situations, and centrally, according to Thomas, to act well in the face of death.

Disasters

According to the International Federation of the Red Cross and Red Crescent Societies, a *disaster* is defined as follows:

> A disaster is a sudden, calamitous event that seriously disrupts the functioning of a community or society and causes human, material, and economic or environmental losses that exceed the community's or society's ability to cope using its own resources. Though often caused by nature, disasters can have human origins. (www.ifrc.org/en/what-we-do/disaster-management/about-disasters/what-is-a-disaster)

Similarly, 'critical incidents' are of particular interest in the NHS:

> Serious Incidents in health care are adverse events, where the consequences to patients, families and carers, staff or organisations are so significant or the potential for learning is so great, that a heightened level of response is justified. (NHS England, 2015)

Designing a community and national disaster response plan will require multidisciplinary collaboration at the highest and, perhaps, unprecedented levels (Ricciardi, 2002).

Aristotelian virtues also come into play in the decision not to treat in a disaster. It takes courage to make an ethical decision that a patient cannot be saved and that the resources both in manpower and equipment are better used in some other area. Disaster triage dictates that the most seriously injured are left to the end – and may even remain untreated – so that those who can be saved can be cared for.

The utilitarian concept of the greatest good for the greatest number is the approach that Mill (1867) used as a functional basis of his ethics. Disaster triage is an example of where the utilitarian rule applies in healthcare. The greater good rule can be justified because of the clear necessity for allocation of resources to benefit the most people (University of Washington School of Medicine, 1998). The physician must show all patients compassion and respect for their dignity, for example by separating them from others and administering appropriate pain relief and sedatives (Geale, 2012).

It is insightful to watch courage in practice in 'disaster scenarios'. The Great East Japan Earthquake on 11 March 2011 caused considerable loss of life and the destruction of livelihood and infrastructure. Linked to this event, but not its cause, was the meltdown and radioactive contamination of the environment from Fukushima Dai-ichi power plant. Noto and colleagues (2013), in this issue on nurses' role in nuclear disaster, open a revealing window as to what happened from the perspective of those who were on the ground, coping with a situation that no one had ever expected to happen, and in which no resources in terms of disaster planning were available. Their account narrates for us the actions of nurses, physicians, paramedical staff and faculty as they volunteered to help and placed themselves at risk in a situation that was, and still is, very unclear as to its consequences. The risk of severe stress reactions increases if the situation that arises from the catastrophe is vast and if there are limited possibilities for individuals to exert any influence (Roxberg et al., 2010). The meaning of courage is also vividly provided in the autobiographies of survivors of the 2004 Indian Ocean tsunami (Roxberg et al., 2010).

Moral courage

From all accounts thus far, it remains unclear quite how many types of courage exist.

Distinctions between physical courage, shown in physically dangerous situations, and moral courage, shown when standing up to others for what is right, have a lengthy history. Lopez and colleagues (2003) suggested that there were three types of courage: physical, moral and vital. However, this categorisation or division is based on reviews of previous studies of courage in specific pre-defined contexts.

Physical courage involves the attempted maintenance of societal good by the expression of physical behaviour grounded in the pursuit of socially valued goals (e.g. a paramedic treating a patient in a collapsed building, or a fire fighter). The definition of 'physical courage' provides inroads into the concept that you can have 'too much' courage, for example:

> Fear of violent harm and death is a natural response to dangerous situations, and so courage requires conquering this fear and overriding the impulse to save oneself through flight or hiding.

Men were not praised for courage when they were unaware of risks; rather, courage meant perceiving the danger and yet still acting in the dangerous but unselfish fashion. Conquering fear required affect regulation, and performing well in battle (as opposed to running away) required behavioral regulation. Thus, again, self-control was involved at two levels. (Baumeister and Exline, 1999: 1175)

Vital courage refers to perseverance through a disease or disability, even when the outcome is ambiguous (e.g. a child with a heart transplant maintaining his or her intensive treatment regimen even though the prognosis is uncertain).

Further support for the physical, moral and vital division was proposed in a literature review and research study conducted by O'Byrne and colleagues (2000). In this research, five open-ended and five scaled questions were administered to 38 participants. The researchers selected and identified major themes in the responses. However, although some responses could be classified into one of the three proposed categories, others were not so easily categorised. *Psychological courage*, as Putnam (1997) described it, is strength in facing one's destructive habits. This form of vital courage may be quite common in that we all struggle with psychological challenges in the forms of stress, sadness and dysfunctional or unhealthy relationships. In light of these threats to our psychological stabilities, we stand up to our dysfunctions by restructuring our beliefs or systematically desensitising ourselves to the fears.

Lord Moran, a former president of the Royal College of Physicians, was a close friend of and personal physician to Winston Churchill, and as such he personally witnessed the atrocities of both World War I and World War II. Moran believed that courage was found on the battlefield, but it was a virtue that everyone was capable of possessing and was not nearly as exclusive as the Aristotelian idea of the 'courageous man'. Lord Moran's famous 'Anatomy of courage' is an essay on the nature of courage in fighting, illustrated in a diary which he kept as a battalion medical officer in the war of 1914–18. 'Courage', writes Lord Moran, 'is a moral quality'. Later he writes, 'Courage is will power'. Bandura (2002: 102) comments:

In the development of a moral self, individuals adopt standards of right and wrong that serve as guides and deterrents for conduct. In this self-regulatory process, people monitor their conduct and the conditions under which it occurs, judge it in relation to their moral standards and perceived circumstances, and regulate their actions by the consequences they apply to themselves. They do things that give them satisfaction and a sense of self-worth.

Courage is necessary in order to deal with everyday fears, and is required extensively in the nursing profession, particularly in situations where the competence of others requires challenge. It takes moral courage to stand up to the norms of a particular organisation or culture. Moral courage is a means to overcome fear through practical action. Knowing one's professional and ethical obligations and personal values is not the same as expressing and acting on those obligations and core values.

We will discuss one particular type of courage much in this book – particularly in Chapter 2 ('Courage to care') and Chapter 5 ('Courage to challenge').

Moral courage is a subtype of prosocial behaviour (e.g. Bierhoff, 2002). Prosocial behaviour 'covers a broad range of actions intended to benefit one or more people' (Batson, 1998: 282), such as helping, showing moral courage, sharing or donating. There is, however, a growing body of evidence pertaining to the costs and moral aspects of prosocial behaviour, particularly in the case of moral courage, a costlier type of prosocial behaviour. For instance, a person who supports a colleague who presses for investigation into possible corporate corruption may do so despite the risk of losing his job. Morally courageous individuals act according to their moral standards, despite the risk of negative financial or professional repercussions (Niesta Kayser et al., 2010).

Moral courage is a willingness to take a stand in defence of principle or conviction even when others do not (Miller, 2000). People who exhibit moral courage are often subject to a number of risks associated with taking a stand, including inconvenience, unpopularity, ostracism, disapproval, derision, and even harm to themselves or their kin (Kidder, 2005). Based on their own research and already existing definitions, Greitemeyer and colleagues (2006) define moral courage as brave behaviour accompanied by anger and indignation which intends to enforce societal and ethical norms without considering one's own social costs. Social costs (such as negative social consequences) distinguish moral courage from other prosocial behaviours.

Cavanagh and Moberg (1999) suggest that moral courage entails the consideration of right and wrong with a conscious choice for moral good. But moral courage is not merely an automatic behaviour per se; it is a practice, consistently doing what one knows one ought to do (Solomon, 1999). It is, however, important not to confuse moral courage with moral arrogance and moral certitude (moral certainty). Moral arrogance involves truly believing that one's own moral stand or judgement is the only correct option regarding a controversial issue, even though others consider differing moral decisions or judgements to be morally acceptable (Gert et al., 2006). Lachman (2007: 256) warns that:

> The personal cost in this case could be loss of employment, if the nurse failed to follow organisational policy. Initially the decision to make this sacrifice may be mingled with angst about unemployment, but such distress is eventually replaced by the sense of peace that comes from acting on a non-negotiable principle.

The acronym CODE is a helpful aid for remembering the underpinnings necessary for moral courage. It also serves as a reminder of the professional obligations of nurses as outlined in the *Code for Ethics for Nurses with Interpretative Statements* (American Nurses Association [ANA], 2001):

Courage to be moral requires:

Obligations to honour (What is the right thing to do?)

Danger to manage (What do I need to handle my fear and uncertainty?)

Expression and action (What action is needed to meet my obligations to the patient and to maintain my integrity?)

Moral distress

The American Nurses Association's *Code of Ethics for Nurses* defines moral distress as 'the condition of knowing the morally right thing to do, but institutional, procedural or social constraints make doing the right thing nearly impossible; it threatens core values and moral integrity' (American Nurses Association, 2015). Action borne out of moral dilemmas in practice might include, for example: taking responsibility for, and arguing for, a preferred decision; advocating on behalf of service users even in the face of hostility and opposition; assertively arguing to deviate from agency procedures or cultural norms; and representing concerns and alternatives to management (Fenton, 2016). These actions are in contrast to practice that is characterised by allegiance to the agency and following procedures. Morley and Macfarlane (2014: 352) found that critical reflection in social work education impacted positively on students developing moral courage, and feeling a sufficient sense of personal agency to take action against injustice.

The term 'moral distress' was first coined by the nurse-philosopher Andrew Jameton and was defined as the negative experience 'when one knows the right thing to do, but institutional constraints make it nearly impossible to pursue the right course of action' (1984: 6). Since this definition, the characteristics and causes of moral distress have been studied and refined by several researchers (McCarthy and Deady, 2008). Webster and Baylis (2003: 208) define moral distress as 'situations in which nurses cannot fulfil their ethical obligations and commitments, thus they fail to pursue what they believe to be the right course of action'.

Moral distress does not have its sole jurisdiction in nurses, however. Moral distress has serious ramifications for all clinicians since it can lead to professional burnout, physical and emotional distress, moral apathy and even leaving the profession (e.g. Pauly et al., 2012). Addressing moral distress is imperative because it can reduce its negative consequences, preserves the moral sensitivity of clinicians and promotes moral courage, which can ultimately promote safe and quality patient care (Escolar-Chua, 2016).

Numerous examples of moral distress emerge in everyday clinical practice, including continued life support, even when it may not be in the best interests of the patient; inadequate communication about end-of-life care among providers, patients and families; inappropriate use of healthcare resources; inadequate staffing; and false hope given to patients and families (Savel and Munro, 2015). The main features that distinguish moral distress from other constructs, such as emotional distress, burnout or post-traumatic stress, are the perceived violation of one's own professional integrity and obligations and the concurrent feeling of being constrained from taking the ethically appropriate action (Epstein and Hamric, 2009). The most detailed definition of moral distress is perhaps that of Judith Wilkinson (1989), who enriched the concept by dealing with pressure. The author mainly claims that an actual or long-term experience of morally distressed nurses is very individual. A clinician must be able to recognise a situation as a moral (or more generally, ethical) problem and come to be convinced that the consequences of such a situation are their co-/responsibility.

Repeated episodes of moral distress can cause health and social care professionals to become disengaged and emotionally traumatised. The impact on the individual is also felt by the rest of the healthcare team, negatively impacting the quality and safety of patient care (Musto et al., 2015). Even when organisations have policies protecting against retaliation for individuals who report wrongdoing, some of these fears are not unfounded. Many who speak out while their colleagues keep quiet do suffer negative consequences of one sort or another. To speak out takes courage. As healthcare organisations work to improve the protection of those who speak out about non-compliance with policies and regulations, it is important to recognise that doing this is only one half of what needs to be done to support moral courage.

Courage also cuts across the training of student health professionals. Courage can be seen as the ability of students to confront their fear of the personal emotional consequences of engaging in what seems the morally right action, as compassionate practice, and can thereby protect against the potential to abandon the professional ideal of compassion. Students can also learn the importance of individual moral responsibility alongside the need for moral support from leaders and role models within the healthcare environment (Curtis, 2014). Also, failing a student in the final placement means standing up to the feelings associated with the experience and having the courage to fail because it is the right thing to do, even when it goes against the cultural norms and apparent culture of failure to fail. It takes courage to speak out and do what is right; courage is the ability to conquer the fear of doing so (Black et al., 2014).

Corley (2002) posits that *moral residue* remains on an individual. This residue may manifest itself in the form of physical symptoms, such as hypertension, ulcers, fatigue and exhaustion, and/or emotional symptoms, sadness, isolation and poor dietary choices, and may result in continued objections/argumentativeness, poor communication, unsafe or poor quality of patient care, detachment from patients or the job, absenteeism, lack of trust and increasing percentages of staff attrition (Prestia et al., 2017). The consequences of managerial moral distress on an organisation have not been clearly described in the literature. Mitton and colleagues (2010) surmise that moral distress and how managers respond to it have negative consequences for healthcare organisations. However, little is known about how ethical dilemmas, which may cause moral distress, are navigated in everyday practice (Pauly et al., 2012).

We will return to 'moral residue' in Chapter 5 in discussing the courage 'to live and die'.

The professional 'duty of candour'

Ethics, law and regulation are found in different orbits circling organisational culture. Organisational leadership and culture play a vital role in cultivating organisational trust, empowering culture that facilitates learning (rather than blame), and nurturing compassion in staff (Wah, 2015). Severe and enduring patient distress can occur in response to neglect – even when unintentional, misdiagnosis, surgical errors and/or deficits in the quality of care occur. An emphasis on the duty of candour has increased awareness of the importance of honesty and acknowledgement of adverse events or 'near misses' in the healthcare setting, in improving the relationship between patients and healthcare professionals (Kenward, 2017). All healthcare professionals have a duty of candour – a professional responsibility to be honest with patients when things go wrong. This is described in *The Professional Duty of Candour*, which introduces this guidance and forms part of a joint statement from eight regulators of healthcare professionals in the UK (see: www.gmc-uk.org/DoC_guidance_english.pdf_61618688.pdf).

Every healthcare professional must be open and honest with patients when something that goes wrong with their treatment or care causes, or has the potential to cause, harm or distress. This means that healthcare professionals must:

- tell the patient (or, where appropriate, the patient's advocate, carer or family) when something has gone wrong
- apologise to the patient (or, where appropriate, the patient's advocate, carer or family)
- offer an appropriate remedy or support to put matters right (if possible)
- explain fully to the patient (or, where appropriate, the patient's advocate, carer or family) the short and long term effects of what has happened.

In the next chapter, a 'courage to care' is discussed where further and wider issues come to the fore.

References

Adler, N.J. and Hansen, H. (2012) 'Daring to care: Scholarship that supports the courage of our convictions', *Journal of Management Inquiry*, 21(2): 128–139.

Ainslie, G. (1975) 'Specious reward: A behavioral theory of impulsiveness and impulse control', *Psychological Bulletin*, 82: 463–496.

Aitamaa, E., Leino-Kilpi, H., Iltanen, S. and Suhonen, R. (2016) 'Ethical problems in nursing management: The views of nurse managers', *Nursing Ethics*, 23(6): 646–658.

Alvey, J.E. (2011) 'The foundations of the ethical tradition of economics: Plato's Republic', *International Journal of Social Economics*, 38(10): 824–846.

American Nurses Association (2001) *Code for Ethics for Nurses with Interpretative Statements*. Silver Spring, MD: American Nurses Publishing.

American Nurses Association (2015) *Code of Ethics for Nurses with Interpretive Statements*. Silver Spring, MD: American Nurses Association. p. 44. Available at: (www.nursingworld. org/codeofethics (accessed 24 May 2018).

Bandura, A. (2002) 'Selective moral disengagement in the exercise of moral agency', *Journal of Moral Education, 31*(2): 101–119.

Batson, C. D. (1998) 'Altruism and prosocial behavior', in D. T. Gilbert, S. T. Fiske and G. Lindzey (eds), *Handbook of Social Psychology* (4th ed., Vol. 2). New York: McGraw Hill. pp. 282–316.

Baumeister, R.F. and Exline, J.J. (1999) 'Virtue, personality, and social relations: Self-control as the moral muscle', *Journal of Personality, 67*(6): 1165–1194.

Bechara, A., Damasio, H., Damasio, A.R. and Lee, G.P. (1999) 'Different contributions of the human amygdala and ventromedial prefrontal cortex to decision-making', *Journal of Neuroscience, 19*(13): 5473–5481.

Bierhoff, H.-W. (2002) *Prosocial Behavior*. New York: Psychology Press.

Black, S., Curzio, J. and Terry, L. (2014) 'Failing a student nurse: A new horizon of moral courage', *Nursing Ethics, 21*(2): 224–238.

Bleakley, A., Marshall, R. and Levine, D. (2014) 'He drove forward with a yell: Anger in medicine and Homer', *The Journal of Medical Humanities, 40*(1): 22–30.

Bournes, D. A. (2002) 'Having courage: A lived experience of human becoming', *Nursing Science Quarterly, 15*(3): 220–229.

Cavanagh, G.F. and Moberg, D.J. (1999) 'The virtue of courage within the organization', in M.L. Pava and P. Primeaus (eds), *Research in Ethical Issues in Organizations*, Vol. 1. Greenwich, CT: JAI Press.

Cleary, S.R. and Doyle, K.E. (2015) 'Whistleblowing need not occur if internal voices are heard: From deaf effect to hearer courage – Comment on "Cultures of silence and cultures of voice: The role of whistleblowing in healthcare organisations"'. *International Journal of Health Policy Management, 5*(1): 59–61.

Corley, M.C. (2002) 'Nurse moral distress: A proposed theory and research agenda', *Nursing Ethics, 9*(6): 636–650.

Crigger, N. and Godfrey, N. (2011) 'Of courage and leaving safe harbors', *Advances in Nursing Science, 34*(4): E13–22.

Curtis, K. (2014) 'Learning the requirements for compassionate practice: Student vulnerability and courage', *Nursing Ethics, 21*(2): 210–223.

Davidson, P.M., Daly, J. and Hill, M.N. (2013) 'Editorial: Looking to the future with courage, commitment, competence and compassion', *Journal of Clinical Nursing, 22*(19–20): 2665–2667.

Dierksmeier, C. and Celano, A. (2012) 'Thomas Aquinas on Justice as a Global Virtue in Business', *Business Ethics Quarterly, 22*(2): 247–272.

Drucker, P.F. (1973) *Management: Tasks, Responsibilities, Practices*. New York, NY: Harper & Row Publishers.

Easmon, C. (2014) 'People matter: Tomorrow's workforce for tomorrow's world', *London Journal of Primary Care, 6*(3): 46–54.

Epstein, E.G. and Hamric, A.B. (2009) 'Moral distress, moral residue, and the crescendo effect', *The Journal of Clinical Ethics, 20*(4): 330–342.

Escolar-Chua, R.L. (2016) 'Moral sensitivity, moral distress, and moral courage among baccalaureate Filipino nursing students', *Nursing Ethics*, 29 June.

Fenton, J. (2016) 'Organisational professionalism and moral courage: Contradictory concepts in social work?', *Critical and Radical Social Work, 4*(2): 199–215.

Finfgeld, D.L. (1999) 'Courage as a process of pushing beyond the struggle', *Qualitative Health Research*, 9(6): 803–814.

Foxall, G.R. (2014) 'Cognitive requirements of competing neuro-behavioral decision systems: Some implications of temporal horizon for managerial behavior in organizations', *Frontiers in Human Neuroscience*, 8: 184.

Geale, S.K. (2012) 'The ethics of disaster management', *Disaster Prevention and Management: An International Journal*, 21(4): 445–462.

Gert, B., Culver, C. and Clouser, K. (2006) *Bioethics: A Systematic Approach* (2nd edn). New York, NY: Oxford University Press.

Glazer, M.P. and Glazer, P.M. (1999) 'On the trail of courageous resistance', *Sociological Inquiry*, 69(2): 276–295.

Greitemeyer, T., Fischer, P., Kastenmüller, A. and Frey, D. (2006) 'Civil courage and helping behaviour: Differences and similarities', *European Psychologist*, 11: 90–98.

Gupta, R., Koscik, T.R., Bechara, A. and Tranel, D. (2011) 'The amygdala and decision-making', *Neuropsychologia*, 49(4): 760–766.

Hannah, S.T., Sweeney, P.J. and Lester, P.B. (2007) 'Toward a courageous mind set: The subjective act and experience of courage', *The Journal of Positive Psychology*, 2: 129–135.

Harvey, J., Erdos, G. and Turnbull, L. (2010) 'How do we perceive heroes?', *Journal of Risk Research*, 12: 313–327.

Hawkins, S.F. and Morse, J. (2014) 'The praxis of courage as a foundation for care', *Journal of Nursing Scholarship*, 46(4): 263–270.

Hecht, D. (2013) 'The neural basis of optimism and pessimism', *Experimental Neurobiology*, 22(3): 173–199.

Hernandez, M. (2008) 'Promoting stewardship behavior in organizations: A leadership model', *Journal of Business Ethics*, 80(1): 121–128.

Houser, R.E. (2002) 'The virtue of courage', in S.J. Pope (ed.), *The Ethics of Aquinas*. Washington, DC: Georgetown University Press. pp. 304–320.

Hu, X., Uhle, F., Fliessbach, K., Wagner, M., Han, Y., Weber, B. and Jessen, F. (2017) 'Reduced future-oriented decision making in individuals with subjective cognitive decline: A functional MRI study', *Alzheimers Dement (Amst)*, 6: 222–231.

Iles, V. (2016) 'Dying is the most grown-up thing we ever do: But do health care professionals prevent us from taking it seriously?', *Health Care Analysis*, 24(2): 105–118.

Jameton, A. (1984) *Nursing Practice: The Ethical Issue*. Englewood Cliffs, NJ: Prentice Hall.

Janis, I.L. (1982) *Groupthink* (2nd edn). Boston: Houghton Mifflin.

Jenson, E. (1997) *Disaster Management Ethics (Training Program)*. Available at: (www.disaster-info.net/lideres/spanish/mexico/biblio/eng/doc13980.pdf (accessed 24 May 2018).

Jones, D.A. (2015) 'Human dignity in healthcare: A virtue ethics approach', *The New Bioethics*, 21(1): 87–97.

Judiciary of England and Wales (2017) *Decision and Short Reasons to be Released to the Media in the Case of Charlie Gard*. Available at: www.judiciary.gov.uk/wp-content/uploads/2017/04/gard-press-summary-20170411.pdf (accessed February 2018).

Kaba, A., Wishart, I., Fraser, K., Coderre, S. and McLaughlin, K. (2016) 'Are we at risk of groupthink in our approach to teamwork interventions in health care?', *Medical Education*, 50(4): 400–408.

Kable, J.W. and Levy, I. (2015) 'Neural markers of individual differences in decision-making', *Current Opinion in Behavioral Sciences*, 5: 100–107.

Kenward, L. (2017) 'Understanding and responding to severe and enduring patient distress resulting from episodes of healthcare', *Nursing Standards*, 31(31): 54–63.

Kidder, R.M. (2005) *Moral Courage: Taking Action When Your Values Are Put to the Test*. New York: HarperCollins.

Klüver, H. and Bucy, P.C. (1939) 'Preliminary analysis of functions of the temporal lobes in monkeys', *Archives of Neurology and Psychiatry*, 42(6): 979–1000.

Kobasa, S.C. (1979) 'Personality and resistance to illness', *American Journal of Community Psychology*, 7: 413–423. Available at: http://dx.doi.org/10.1007/BF00894383 (accessed 24 May 2018).

Kurzynski, M. (2012) 'Peter Drucker: Modern day Aristotle for the business community', *Journal of Management History*, 18(1): 6–23.

Lachman, V.D. (2007) 'Moral courage in action: case studies', *Medsurg Nursing*, 16(4): 275– 277.

Ladikos, A. (2004) 'Revisiting the virtue of courage in Aristotle', *Phronimon*, 5(2): 77–92.

Likona, T. (1991) *Educating for Character*. New York, NY: Bantam Books.

Lima, S.L. and Bednekoff, P.A. (1999) 'Temporal variation in danger drives antipredator behavior: The predation risk allocation hypothesis', *The American Naturalist, 153*: 649–659.

Lindh, I.B., Barbosa da Silva, A., Berg, A. and Severinsson, E. (2010) 'Courage and nursing practice: A theoretical analysis', *Nursing Ethics*, 17(5): 551–565.

Lopez, S.J., O'Byrne, K.K. and Peterson, S. (2003) 'Profiling courage', in S.J. Lopez and C.R. Snyder (eds), *Positive Psychological Assessment: A Handbook of Models and Measures*. Washington, DC: American Psychological Association. pp. 185–197.

Magnano, P., Paolillob, A., Plataniac, S. and Giuseppe Santisic, G. (2017) 'Courage as a potential mediator between personality and coping', *Personality and Individual Differences, 111*: 13–18.

McCarthy, J. and Deady, R. (2008) 'Moral distress reconsidered', *Nursing Ethics, 15*(2): 254–262.

McMillan, T.M. and Rachman, S.J. (1988) 'Fearlessness and courage in paratroopers undergoing training', *Personality and Individual Differences*, 2: 373–378.

Mill, J.S. (1867) *Utilitarianism* (3rd edn). London: Longmans, Green, Reader and Dyer.

Miller, W.I. (2000) *The Mystery of Courage*. Cambridge, MA: Harvard University Press.

Mitton, C., Peacock, S., Storch, J., Smith, N. and Cornelissen, E. (2010) 'Moral distress among healthcare managers: Conditions, consequences and potential responses', *Health Policy*, 6(2): 99–112.

Mobbs, D. and Kim, J.J. (2015) 'Neuroethological studies of fear, anxiety, and risky decision-making in rodents and humans', *Current Opinion in Behavioral Sciences*, 5: 8–15.

Morley, C. and Macfarlane, S. (2014) 'Critical social work as ethical social work: Using critical reflection to research students' resistance to neoliberalism', *Critical and Radical Social Work*, 2(3): 337–355.

Mowrer, O.H. (1960) *Learning Theory and Behavior*. New York: Wiley.

Muris, P. (2009) 'Fear and courage in children: Two sides of the same coin?', *Journal of Child and Family Studies*, 18(4): 486–490.

Murray, J.S. (2010) 'Letter to the editor', *Nursing Outlook*, 58: 6–7.

Musto, L.C., Rodney, P.A. and Vanderheide, R. (2015) 'Toward interventions to address moral distress: Navigating structure and agency', *Nursing Ethics*, 22(1): 91–102.

Naylor, C.D. and Naylor, K.T. (2012) 'Seven provocative principles for health care reform', *Journal of the American Medical Association, 307*: 919–920.

NHS England (2013) *Care, Compassion, Competence, Communication, Courage, Commitment. Compassion in Practice. One Year On*. Available at: www.england.nhs.uk/wp-content/uploads/2016/05/cip-one-year-on.pdf (accessed 29 May 2018).

NHS (2014) *Briefing Note: Issues Highlighted by the 2014 NHS Staff Survey in England.* Twelfth annual national survey of NHS staff. Oxford.

NHS England (2015) *Serious Incident Framework: Supporting Learning to Prevent Recurrence.* Available at: www.england.nhs.uk/wp-content/uploads/2015/04/serious-incidnt-framwrk-upd.pdf (accessed 29 May 2018).

Niesta Kayser, D., Greitemeyer, T., Fischer, P. and Frey, D. (2010) 'Why mood affects help giving, but not moral courage: Comparing two types of prosocial behaviour', *European Journal of Social Psychology*, December: 1136–1157.

Nili, U., Goldberg, H., Weizman, A. and Dudai, Y. (2010) 'Fear thou not: Activity of frontal and temporal circuits in moments of real-life courage', *Neuron*, 66(6): 949–962.

Norton, P.J. and Weiss, B.J. (2009) 'The role of courage on behavioral approach in a fear-eliciting situation: A proof-of-concept pilot study', *Journal of Anxiety Disorders*, 23: 212–217.

Noto, Y., Kitamiya, C., Itaki, C., Urushizaka, M., Kidachi, R. and Yamabe, H. (2013) 'Role of nurses in a nuclear disaster: Experience in the Fukushima Dai-ichi nuclear power plant accident', *International Nursing Review*, 60(2): 196–200.

O'Byrne, K.K., Lopez, S.J. and Petersen, S. (2000) 'Building a theory of courage: A precursor to change?', paper presented at the 108th Annual Convention of the American Psychological Association, Washington, DC, August.

Pachur, T., Mata, R. and Hertwig, R. (2017) 'Who dares, who errs? Disentangling cognitive and motivational roots of age differences in decisions under risk', *Psychological Science*, 28(4): 504–518.

Palmer, P.J. (1990) *The Active Life: A Spirituality of Work, Creativity and Caring.* New York, NY: Harper & Row.

Pauly, B.M., Varcoe, C. and Storch, J. (2012) 'Framing the issues: Moral distress in health care', *HEC Forum*, 24: 1–11.

Perugini, M. and Bagozzi, R.P. (2004) 'The distinction between desires and intentions', *European Journal of Social Psychology*, 34(1): 69–84.

Peterson, C. and Seligman, M.E.P. (2004) *Character Strengths and Virtues: A Handbook and Classification.* Washington, DC: American Psychological Association.

Plato (1973) *Laches and Charmides.* New York: Bobbs-Merrill.

Prestia, A.S., Sherman, R.O. and Demezier, C. (2017) 'Chief Nursing Officers' experiences with moral distress', *Journal of Nursing Administration*, 47(2): 101–107.

Pury, C.L.S., Kowalski, R.M. and Spearman, M.J. (2007) 'Distinctions between general and personal courage', *Journal of Positive Psychology*, 2: 99–114.

Putnam, D. (1997) 'Psychological courage', *Philosophy, Psychiatry and Psychology*, 4: 1–11.

Rachman, S. (1994) 'The overprediction of fear: A review', *Behaviour Research and Therapy*, 32(7): 683–690.

Rachman, S. J. (1984) 'Fear and courage', *Behavior Therapy*, 15: 109–120.

Rachman, S. J. (2004) 'Fear and courage: A psychological perspective', *Social Research*, 71: 149–176.

Raffel, S. (2011) 'The interplay of courage and reason in moral action', *History of the Human Sciences*, 24(5): 89–102.

Rate, C.R. (2010) 'Defining the features of courage: A search for meaning', in C.L.S. Purt and S.J. Lopez (eds), *Courage: Modern Research on an Ancient Virtue.* Washington, DC: American Psychological Association.

Rate, C.R., Clarke, J.A., Lindsay, D.R. and Sternberg, R.J. (2007) 'Implicit theories of courage', *The Journal of Positive Psychology*, 2: 80–98.

Reardon, K.K. (2007) 'Courage as a skill', *Harvard Business Review*, 85: 58–64.

Ricciardi, R. (2002) 'Disaster preparedness – the courage to respond', *Journal of Pediatric Health Care*, 16(5): 211–212.

Roxberg, A., Sameby, J., Brodin, S., Fridlund, B. and da Silva, A.B. (2010) 'Out of the wave: The meaning of suffering and relief from suffering as described in autobiographies by survivors of the 2004 Indian Ocean tsunami', *International Journal of Qualitative Studies on Health and Well-being*, 5(3) doi: 10.3402/qhw.v5i3.5323.

Sadooghiasl, A., Parvizy, S. and Ebadi, A. (2016) 'Concept analysis of moral courage in nursing: A hybrid model', *Nursing Ethics*, 20 April: 6–19.

Sarros, J.C., Cooper, B.K. and Hartican, A.M. (2006) 'Leadership and character', *Leadership & Organization Development Journal*, 27(8): 682–699.

Savel, R.H. and Munro, C.L. (2015) 'Moral distress, moral courage', *American Journal of Critical Care*, 24(4): 276–278.

Schilpzand, P., Hekman, D. and Mitchell, T. (2014) 'An inductively-generated typology and process model of workplace courage', *Organization Science*, 26(1): 52–77.

Shelp, E.E. (1984) 'Courage: A neglected virtue in the patient–physician relationship', *Social Science & Medicine*, 18: 351–360.

Shepela, S.T. (1999) 'Courageous resistance – a special case of altruism', *Theory and Psychology*, 9: 787–805.

Solomon, R.C. (1999) *A Better Way to Think about Business: How Personal Integrity Leads to Corporate Success*. New York: Oxford University Press.

Tjeltveit, A.C. (2003) 'Implicit virtues, divergent goods, multiple communities', *American Behavioral Scientist*, 47(4): 395–414.

University of Washington School of Medicine (1998) *Ethics in Medicine*. Available at: https://depts.washington.edu/bioethx (accessed 29 May 2018).

Wah, T.M. (2015) 'Cultivating duty of candour requires organisational leadership and culture', BMJ, *351*: h4123.

Webster, G. and Baylis, F. (2003) 'Ethical distress in health care environments', *Ethics in practice for registered nurses*, Canadian Nurses Association, October 2003 (available at https://www.cna-aiic.ca/~/media/cna/page-content/pdf-en/ethics_pract_ethical_distress_oct_2003_e.pdf).

Wilkinson, J.M. (1989) 'Moral distress in nursing practice: A labour and delivery nurse's experience', *Journal of Obstetric, Gynecologic and Neonatal Nursing*, 23(1): 16–29.

Woodard, C. (2004) 'Hardiness and the concept of courage', *Consulting Psychology Journal: Practice and Research*, 56(3): 173–185.

Woodard, C.R. and Pury, C.L.S. (2007) 'The construct of courage: Categorization and measurement', *Consulting Psychology Journal: Practice and Research*, 59: 135–147.

Yechiam, E., Druyan, M. and Ert, E. (2008) 'Observing others' behavior and risk taking in decisions from experience', *Judgment and Decision Making*, 3: 493–500.

Zagzebski, L.T. (1996) *Virtues of the Mind: An Inquiry into the Nature of Virtue and the Ethical Foundations of Knowledge*. Cambridge, UK: Cambridge University Press.

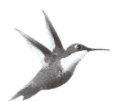

COURAGE TO CARE

REBECCA MYERS

Introduction

Courage to care and courage in being a carer are quite profoundly different things. This chapter is about the 'courage to care'. It does take courage to care, to open your heart and react with sympathy or compassion or indignation or enthusiasm when it is easier – and sometimes safer – not to get involved. But people who take the risk, who deliberately discard a shield of indifference, make a tremendous discovery: 'It does take courage to care, the more things you care about, and the more intensely you care, the more alive you become' – Earl Nightingale.

To care for another requires you to become emotionally involved. Being emotionally involved can mean you are vulnerable and get hurt. This is why it takes courage to care. But if you believe that a central tenet of care is not just what you *do to* someone but how you care *about* them as a fellow human being, it is impossible not to 'get involved'.

Who cares and how?

Whilst care is often seen as a 'transaction' between carer and recipient, it is clear that there is a much wider culture of care. This culture of care indeed varies across different cultures. Professional carers (a group which includes all health and social work professionals) are subject to constraints in time and finances, which may compromise their ability to care, and these can also be particularly pertinent for unpaid carers (which includes family and friends).

It is important to distinguish between caring and the role that professionals play in delivering 'care' which, from the outside, can look similar, but will not show the medical and nursing theories and professional thought processes that are informing the professional's types of interventions. This is because the courage required in these circumstances will be very different. Working as a health professional requires one to have a standard of knowledge and ethical practice in a therapeutic and professional relationship.

Thus, whilst a carer and a professional may be carrying out the same 'task', and may demonstrate the same level of empathy and sensitivity, the knowledge applied to the tasks are most likely to be executed rather differently and, in most cases, of a higher level due to the professional's training. This is important to state as it high-lights why courage required on behalf of the professional is different to that of the carer, and in particular the family carer. Being aware of the underlying pathology and thus associated risks to health and wellbeing brings different challenges to caring for a loved one where your knowledge in these areas may be less extensive. In his book, *When Doctors Become Patients*, Robert Klitzman (2007) explores the experience of over 70 doctors as they face the other side of medicine and recounts their struggle with both knowing the prognosis of their conditions, the risk of medical error and the realisation of the limitations of medical interventions. This book builds on what Jung called the phenomenon of 'wounded healers'.

The impact of caring

Much research has been done to explore the impact of caring on health profession-als and informal carers. In England, 42% of nurses report feeling burnout (Aiken et al., 2002). Burnout can result in high staff turnover and absenteeism or presentee-ism, resulting in significant financial cost to organisations. In addition, sickness rates in the NHS (average 10.7 days/employee/year) are cited as being significantly higher than those for workers in the private sector (average 6.4 days/employee/year).

Carers UK state that there are over 6.5 million carers in the UK (www.carersuk.org/news-and-campaigns/press-releases/facts-and-figures) with an anticipated increase to 9 million by 2037. People providing high levels of care are twice as likely to be permanently sick or disabled and the impact on them includes financial, social and physical stress.

Valerie Iles (2005) argues that it is difficult to care for others unless we are also capable of caring for ourselves – what she describes as 'caring for our ability to care for others' – so we need to enlarge our definition of care as: 'the will to engage in acts of work and courage in order to nurture another's personal growth and our own ability to do so'. Therefore, healthcare involves acts of courage that enable or promote the flourishing of others and our own ability to flourish in their service.

The experience of one of the authors of this book (RM) is that, as a clinician, when one is able to be 'present' with patients and really listen to what they want from their life and what is needed for them to realise their potential, the interaction creates a sense of joy and purpose. However, when either pressure in the 'system' distracts attention, or there is a 'difficulty' in connecting, even in a non-judgemental way, there is a sense of failure and frustration and disappointment from the patient and the professional. It is the quality of the relationship (and all that that requires) that gives both the professional and the patient a sense of good care.

Evidence of courage

As we discussed in Chapter 1, courage takes many forms, such as Kirsty Broden, the nurse who was killed whilst running to help people in the terrorist attack on London Bridge in 2017. Her response was clearly a courageous act, but we are also interested in the everyday courage required for health professionals to work in an environment of high complexity, responsibility and uncertainty where their knowledge, or ability to control the outcomes, can be limited. Being able to be honest about that both to themselves and to their patients, who often look to them to give hope and cure, and to continue to do this day after day requires a level of moral and emotional courage that rarely gets explored or acknowledged.

Healthcare, and the types of healthcare services and patients cared for, varies enormously with different types of courage being required to be able to give the type of care that has a therapeutic impact. Often the circumstances in which we as health professionals are caring, is against a backdrop of the primary need being more fundamental such as housing, benefits, a job or broken down relationships and loneliness. The ability of health professionals to impact on these things directly can be very difficult and thus to be able, in the face of people's predicament, to just be alongside them can require a lot of emotional courage. This can be equally difficult for colleagues in social care who, whilst working in these areas, are increasingly faced with significant budget cuts and having to make difficult rationing decisions with people with significant needs.

In a recent conference convened at the Nuffield Trust (2018), on reflections 'on the welfare state from primary care', Jonathan Tomlinson, an Inner City General Practitioner based in East London, described how these fundamental unmet needs manifest in his patients' lives and contribute to their physical and mental ill health, leaving him, at times, feeling inadequate and distressed.

This feeling of helplessness or inadequacy is remarkably common, and can be what leads to significant distress for both professional carers and families. But being able to acknowledge the difficulty in this for patients and professionals alike offers an opportunity for them to create a courageous relationship and to be strong and brave together. In reflecting on the last days of her mother's life, Valerie Iles (2016) suggests that facing death honestly in all its rawness might enable us all to be better at dealing with what she describes as 'the most grown up thing' humans will ever do – die.

It is this ability to face and manage our vulnerability that demands of us all to be courageous. In an environment where care involves facing the inevitability of death or, for those with a degenerative disease, the sense sometimes of helplessness, and the associated pull to 'do' something, save them, 'cure' them, it takes courage to confront these emotions in ourselves and sit with this unease rather than dismiss them or avoid them, rather being able to accept things and adjust our expectations and our actions accordingly (Dartington, 2010). We again see this not just as healthcare professionals or colleagues in social care but also as carers of our own families.

Iles (2005) defines 'care' as a 'thinner' and more widely disseminated form of love, taking this as an extension of Scott Peck (1990), in his book *The Road Less Travelled*, who describes love as being an act of work or courage. Thus our ability to 'love' supports us in being able to care. This offers an interesting perspective on the emotional involvement of professionals with their patients/clients but also on the ability to give love. The importance of love will be picked up in Chapter 6 when we explore how this assists in creating the conditions for courage to flourish.

Courage to face our own emotions

Being able to explore death and morbidity in people requires us to have a level of comfort with our own morbidity and mortality. This means being aware of when we are either avoiding or over associating with patient's experiences in a way that is not helpful either to us or to our patients. Drawing on our own experiences and sharing them can help build empathic relationships with people, but can also risk shifting the focus too much on to the professional.

The ability to care requires us to be able to continue to identify with those in our care as individuals and to have both empathy and compassion in our interactions (McPherson et al., 2016). But can you train people to be compassionate or does recruiting people with the 'right' values mean they will be able to sustain that level of emotional availability and compassion to people when working day in and out in healthcare?

The evidence suggests that during the course of training or in early years post qualifying, this diminishes due to the conditions in which people find themselves and in response to their own emotional needs (Smith, 1995; Shapiro, 2008).

Part of this is related to the *socialisation* of professionals and the view that they must suppress their own emotions to give primacy to that of their patients, and yet patients and families repeatedly share how knowing their health professionals are also upset makes them feel 'cared about', not just in receipt of Care. Socialisation is not the only factor and the development of both social and psychological defence mechanisms can be at play to enable individuals to cope with the emotions evoked in their caring experiences (Menzies Lyth, 1988).

In the dynamic of the relationship of kindness between patients and staff, when staff and patients can recognise their shared (*kinship*) experiences of vulnerability or distress, there is the potential to reduce anxiety and defensiveness. When we as health professionals develop some of the common defence mechanisms including displacement, projection, rationalisation and sublimation, these are not necessarily a sign of something being wrong, but can become a problem if under or over used. Without the recognition that we may have developed these, or the space and time to explore them in a supportive and non-judgemental environment, they can impede our capacity (be it the professional or the carer) to care and impact on our own wellbeing (Ballatt and Campling, 2011). When looking at the particular stress for staff and families who are providing care for patients with conditions such as dementia, the behavioural and psychological symptoms can result in staff/carers experiencing physical or verbal abuse, resulting in feeling anxious or stressed (Rodney, 2000). This can add to an already heavy physically demanding workload. This, alongside managing multiple morbidities, places increased intellectual demands on staff as they try to process what is causing distress to the person with dementia and employ strategies to support them.

Attempts to look at what support staff could do to manage their own stress and to stay emotionally connected to their patients have included the use of self-compassion and mindfulness. This needs to be helpful from an individual and organisational level, recognising and removing the barriers to this, including: a lack of time and space to stop and be mindful or self-compassionate; an inability to express emotions at work; and a lack of organisational modelling of compassion in action and professional values which often embody stoicism and are exclusively patient-centred, meaning that staff emotions don't get explored. We shall return to this in Chapter 6.

Accessing these types of interventions requires staff to be able to speak up and acknowledge their own emotions and distress, and for everyone to see this not as an indication of individual failure to cope but as a recognised occupational hazard that is just as risky as exposure to harmful chemicals.

This shift in ability to care, be emotionally present, and thus courageous, is reflected in the work of Maben et al. (2012b), where they look at staff motivation, affect and wellbeing and how they relate to patients' experiences. Their research points to the importance of seven staff variables that correlate positively with patient-reported experience:

- A good local team/workgroup climate
- Co-worker support
- Job satisfaction
- A positive organisational climate
- Organisational support
- Low emotional exhaustion
- Supervisor support.

Emotional 'distress' of carers

Understanding of what various types of interventions support carers is relatively limited often due to a lack of appreciation of the causes that sit underneath their emotional distress. Reasons can range from fear, anger, distress, guilt or even shame. By listening to the attributions carers make about their own role in the situation they find themselves in and being able to sensitively and constructively reflect that back to them offers opportunities for more effective interventions.

In busy clinical environments this can be difficult but working in community settings such as district nursing offers greater opportunity not only to observe how carers are really managing but to engage in a conversation with them that can openly acknowledge the difficulties of what they are doing and how they are coping. With greater numbers of older people looking after their spouses at home, it is not unnatural to see people in their 80s or 90s trying to care for their loved one and not wanting to bother family members or admit they cannot cope for fear of being separated through the need for admission to a care home. Being able to have these conversations sensitively requires not only skill but also courage to confront what is an extremely distressing time for people.

Courage to be honest

The courage to be honest repeatedly surfaces when we look at what is required to raise issues or confront situations and not collude with people about the impact of their own behaviour on their health.

It is critical for health professionals to be able to shift from the traditional paternalistic ways of relating, to adult-to-adult conversations (Berne, 1964) that are respectful and non-judgemental and have the intention of helping people to reach their full potential. Engaging in these types of conversations can run the risk of rejection, anger and complaint as the message may not be popular and may be difficult to hear.

In his book, *Games People Play* (1964), Eric Berne examines the transactions between individuals and describes how social interactions can be a 'game' whereby individuals assume a particular 'role'. This has developed, often at the unconscious level, due to repeated early childhood patterns of relating. These patterns, often not recognised, serve some implicit purpose in communicating both content and the relationship – for example, I am the parent who is encouraging you, the unsure child. This 'transaction' is not only managing communication content but also emotions – for example, I, the parent, am upset that you are anxious and want to reassure you; I, the child, am frightened and need you to make me feel more secure by reassuring me. This is a useful transaction, but at times they can keep people 'stuck' and be unhelpful. Being able to not only recognise your own patterns and those of the other, but to change the patterns in order to shift the relationship into a more constructive dynamic can help both parties to have more honest and courageous conversations.

Courage to stay 'person-centred'

Often in the delivery of healthcare, despite the aspirations, it is the patients or clients who are having to adapt to fit the procedures and structures of health and social care. We see this in headlines where health providers are advising patients not to come to emergency departments or see their GP but to use alternative services to reduce the demand on overstretched facilities, as well as with well-meaning and anxious families who can unintentionally disempower relatives by doing things for them or talking on their behalf.

In environments such as care homes there is a need for courage of staff to face and explore older people's wellbeing and identity near death, as illness, ageing and the dying process affect one's sense of self and identity (Osterland et al., 2016). The management of this transition can have a significant impact on how well cared for people feel and the quality of their life at this stage, as well as how families are supported in what can be an extremely distressing decision. Providing 'identity-promoting' care is important. Part of this is being able to express thoughts and feelings about death, which helps sustain personhood and a meaningful existence at the end of our lives. One of the interesting things to observe is how often staff also feel they have to subordinate themselves to the values and norms of other staff and the residents due to the communal living. Having spent a lifetime developing a sense of who they were and what they wanted or valued in life, it can take courage for staff to push against these rituals and norms (Osterland et al., 2016).

In environments that are highly structured it requires courage of staff to not follow rules and procedures and impose routines that may suit the 'smooth' running of the home, rather than the flexibility and freedom of residents to choose what they do and when. When there is lack of flexibility the 'home' takes on more of an institutional approach which can lead to residents feeling reduced as an individual as decisions are taken away from them and their views not considered. This may be difficult for staff to hear and understand or accept how their behaviour contributes to this, especially if staff feel they have no control over many of these rituals themselves. Part of this institutionalisation occurs where these behaviours become normalised and are not questioned. Campaigns such as 'John's Campaign' (Gerrard and Jones, 2014), which promote open visiting for carers as a way of disrupting this normalisation, can offer insight into how people cope at home and bring a greater sense of the resident or patient's identity, providing alternative perspectives on caring.

Courage to take risks

Adopting risk can be essential to progress, and this needs courage for all concerned.

In the *Professional Standards of Occupational Therapy Practice* published by the College of Occupational Therapists, positive risk is defined as 'recognising and accepting, but managing, risk when there is a positive objective or outcome' (p. xi).

A positive approach to risk, involving courage on the part of those providing care, is argued to be beneficial in a number of scenarios. For example, in the guidance from the Department of Health (2010), *Nothing Ventured, Nothing Gained: Risk Guidance for People with Dementia*, it was argued that 'everyone involved in supporting persons with dementia to take a proportionate, measured and enabling approach to risk'. It had been noted, for example, that one of the biggest barriers to enabling people with dementia to have more control over their lives is an overly cautious approach to risk. A lack of risk engagement might, for example, specifically also act as a barrier to offering people with dementia a full choice of services and support, particularly when accessing personal budgets or self-directed support. Whilst risk is part of the discussion with patients and families in the consenting of procedures, conversations around perceived risks and managing when people are discharged, or decisions by community staff and primary care around admission, are often a less formal part of the process. This managing of risk is a key part of the care which can create significant anxiety for professional staff (and families) and is often less explicitly discussed.

Courage to admit mistakes

In providing care, a core element is that of building a trusting relationship and this includes honesty not just about what is happening, but also about mistakes that may happen. In an environment that prides itself on success and clinical excellence, being able to admit errors both to yourself and to others can be difficult and yet error is part of human fallibility.

Example from Practice 2.1

At the opening of a conference for clinical staff in a medium-sized District General Hospital, staff were asked if they had ever made a mistake. The facilitator raised their hand first and then every person also raised their hand. They were then asked to keep their hand up if they remembered the details of the mistake and the name of the patient involved. All hands remained in the air. What was interesting was the anxiety of the new CEO who had been asked to talk at the conference who later admitted her level of anxiety at seeing the uniformity of the response and the sense of responsibility she felt for these errors.

On the agenda for the conference was one of the most senior consultants who had agreed to speak about their own mistake with a patient when they had first become a consultant. The facilitator had offered on several occasions to talk through the story before the event as a way of supporting the individual but they had declined saying they did not feel the need. When the time came for them to speak they took to the floor and began. When they reached the point at which they shared the patient's response to being told of the error, they became overwhelmed and had to take a moment to recover. The patient had been understandably upset but it was the phrase, 'I trusted you and you let me down' that was the most difficult aspect of their response for the consultant to face.

This was so difficult as it spoke to one of the underlying principles of the professional–patient relationship – trust – and yet the expectation that health professionals do not make any mistakes is clearly unrealistic.

This view (and the psychobiological evidence) of the importance of the relationship between patient and professional is imperative and one that is explored throughout all undergraduate education. Thus action that could damage this is something both health and social care colleagues are fully aware of. This raises an important issue around the psychological contract that is made with health professionals and the organisation. How many members of Boards recognise the courage required for staff to do their work, the barriers to this and the associated impact of not overcoming them, and then build this into health professional employment contracts and working week? Far too often these mitigating conditions are not available and staff, when showing signs of distress, are 'sent' to occupational health departments – often situated at the back of the hospital or off site and not particularly aesthetically designed, which does not give the impression that this is a normal response to the distress and that 'we value you'.

Example from Practice 2.2

Simon was in charge over the weekend and, in doing the allocation for the week ahead, thought that the agency nurse that was booked wouldn't be needed. Discouraged from contacting the team leader at the weekends, he decided to speak to the agency nurse directly to give her plenty of warning and suggested that she might be cancelled but to come in on the Monday as normal and discuss with the team leader. He made a note for the team leader explaining what he'd done and for her to check what she wanted to do. On the Monday whilst out seeing a sick patient he received a call from the team leader shouting at him that he should not have taken that action and that he was in trouble. He explained that he was with a sick patient and was told he would be spoken to when he got back to the office. Already anxious about the patient, he now had additional distress due to the behaviour of the manager. On returning to the office Simon made several attempts to discuss the matter with the manager but they kept avoiding him. The next day Simon made again and apologised to the manager if he had done something wrong and also challenged the manager's behaviour and said, in the context of both staff welfare and patient safety, he felt it was unproductive.

Conditions that add to an already stressful situation due to unhelpful management practices only exacerbate the professional's anxiety. Simon's decision to feedback the impact of the manager's behaviour provided an opportunity for her to see the impact. Speaking out can lead to negative consequences for staff and mechanisms to support those in these situations are important.

Mentoring and supporting people who have displayed moral courage in order to help sustain them and develop resilience are important. We are social animals, and as described in Chapter 1, if speaking out leads to an experience of isolation, people will learn to withhold views, or paradoxically, in the effort to stay in relationships with others, may suppress important and authentic aspects of themselves from these relationships in order to continue to be accepted. This can lead to inauthentic relationships, which limit the growth of both parties, reduce resilience, leading to a range of negative psychological outcomes, and create risk for patients and colleagues if concerns are not raised.

Connecting with others to create supportive relationships that are empathic and able to hear the distress of the person by building a trusting relationship is important. Helping them to process their distress and make sense of their experience in a constructive manner is key. Interventions such as Restorative Justice (see work by Suzanne Shales on the use of Restorative Justice for those who have experienced trauma in their work) enable the person to see vulnerability in others and offer support. Far too often we hear statements such as that staff need to be more resilient. Whilst clearly resilience is important, we would argue that most NHS staff are incredibly resilient and that resilience needs to be reframed from simply an individual to a relational capacity. Normalising their experiences, and enabling others to be 'heard' and their stories acknowledged which validates them and their experiences, is also important. This final point is very much the case with Schwartz Rounds® where staff that are not the most visible, yet carrying out key roles, present on panels about the emotional aspects of their work (Point of Care Foundation, n.d.b). This experience provides a positive impact for these staff and others to hear their stories and confront their own ignorance or understanding prior to hearing them.

This need for support also extends to supporting patients' and carers' experience being heard by those working in healthcare through forums such as NHS England's Carer Network (www.england.nhs.uk/commitment-to-carers/carers-toolkit).

By making others' experiences visible and sharing both positive and difficult emotions it normalises them and reduces the fear of exposure, and thus the need to be courageous.

Difficult conversations

Part of what stops us from taking action is the difficulty in having conversations which are uncomfortable for those involved, due to a range of issues. Within the context of healthcare, these can be in both clinical and organisational situations. Within the clinical context, failure to have the conversations can leave patients and families describing how they feel they were left to face a difficult situation on their own. In their work on developing effective relationships between patients and staff, The Point of Care Foundation shares the experience of Kieran Sweeney (Point of Care Foundation, n.d.a). Kieran was a GP who, following his diagnosis of malignant mesothelioma, identified how the technical aspects of his care were excellent *but* that the team's difficulty in confronting the reality of his situation, and being honest with him, left him feeling isolated and 'devoid of hope':

> Medicine is not solely a technical activity and pursuit, medicine is about understanding and being with people at the edge of the human predicament. Caring for somebody is a transactional activity ... it's the relational care where I've felt that the experience has been less than satisfactory ... my insight is that it doesn't take much to change from upsetting or insensitive communication to communication that puts someone much more at ease.
>
> *Source*: Point of Care Foundation, video available at: www.pointofcare-foundation.org.uk/our-work/ sweeney-programme/. Reproduced here with kind permission of the Point of Care Foundation.

Conversations can be difficult because they are often having to convey a terminal diagnosis and poor prognosis, which in turn reduces the sense of hope and optimism for families (e.g. Meyer, 2014). The skill in having the conversation and getting the balance between being empathic and emotionally available as well as professional and appropriately removed, is an on-going challenge for all practitioners and the introduction of effective communication skills that provide a structure can assist practitioners who often describe how they do not yet know 'how' to have these conversations.

Equipping staff with a structure reduces their anxiety so they are able to be more emotionally available to the patient and family. Practising the use of different phrases, which are more empathic, and being mindful of language to prevent use of clinical jargon or slang is important, alongside the ability to explore professionals' own emotions and reactions to the emotions of others.

The use of 'forum theatre' is increasingly used to enable staff to practise and receive feedback in real time as to how they are approaching the conversation and what it feels like from the recipient's point of view. Finding ways to help patients feed back to staff directly on what it was like to be cared for by them is still undeveloped but needs to be encouraged if we are to achieve a rich and honest way of relating with each other.

Example from Practice 2.3

Harriet, registered nurse

I remember my own experience of waiting with my father to hear about his diagnosis of kidney cancer. Called in to the consultant's office, we could see he was rushed and agitated. He started to talk about having some tests to find out what was happening

(Continued)

(Continued)

which left us both confused. I asked if the previous results were back and if so, did they not show he had cancer? The consultant asked how we knew this. When informed a junior doctor had told us on discharge, the consultant became agitated, saying that we shouldn't have been told by someone who had not undertaken the specialist training in communication skills. Initially shocked and, whilst recognising the consultant was stressed, I fed back that his comments were unhelpful and that the main issue was whether the diagnosis was cancer or not. This feedback made the consultant stop, reflect, apologise and then focus on explaining the results and what they meant.

Being able to say what they were experiencing, and the consultant realising his response was inappropriate, enabled the consultation to shift to a more honest and productive one.

As health professionals we will regularly encounter situations that require courage, but when presented with these situations we will not always respond courageously (Kerfoot, 1999). Courage is the result of a culture of integrity where doing 'the right thing' is required, recognised and rewarded, and that starts with clinical leaders who actively plan and build cultures of courage. (We shall return to this in Chapter 6.) However, courage does not simply just 'appear' instantaneously upon graduating–clinical educators must accept some responsibility for developing on-going educational opportunities for staff to discuss, reflect and practise courage that can be transferred to any clinical or future setting where staff are required to 'do the right thing' (Alpers et al., 2012). A combination of didactic and clinical assignments, as well as simulation, have been proven to be valuable as a way of inculcating the essentiality of courage into practice, creating the expectation that highly emotive conversations are normal and staff are expected to undertake them.

This expectation is internalised by the staff as a collective view and assists them in using the power of the group to build a sense of authority when required to have these difficult conversations (Maxfield et al., 2005). This resonates with one of the author's (RM) own initial training where the role of the nurse was defined as *the patient's advocate when they could not advocate for themselves*. This view, taught over 30 years ago, is still at the core of what they believe is the role of the nurse and is shared and quoted by others who trained at the same institution.

Having a common definition and expected approach enables staff to reflect on what they see in the clinical setting and to question and model this to others. This then becomes 'normal' practice, thus reducing the anxiety that can be encountered. It also highlights when this does not happen as something of note, which can prompt discussion and learning.

The risk of not being courageous in caring

Courage in end-of-life care is particularly important where access to palliative care and hospice input is often not provided as patients, families and, at times, health professionals do not prioritise it. Staff are often torn between the need to provide the best care for patients and families, and creating healthy workplaces for staff which is essential for any caring to occur. (We will encounter courage in dying again in Chapter 4.)

With death often still seen as a failure, it means there is little preparation for this meaningful event in contrast to other life events such as childbirth, where there are plans and informed participants researching options and alternative practices. Even the physical environment for life events for birth, with specially decorated rooms, is often in stark contrast to end-of-life care on a busy ward area with little space or opportunity to attend to the environment as life ends. It requires courage for staff to resist pressure to focus on the curative aspects of care and push for more person-alised care for those who are dying, making the personal, professional and financial case for doing so.

Example from Practice 2.4

Ruth, district nurse

Ruth is a district nurse with over 25 years' experience who has nursed thousands of patients in the end stage of life and developed a level of confidence in supporting patients and families during these difficult times. Over the years she describes how the level of oversight and scrutiny has increased which, whilst it has some advantages, has led to a risk-adverse culture which she argues is not always in the best interest of the patient, but in the best interest of the organisation in terms of risk management.

She is on duty when a call comes from a family who are becoming increasingly frightened as their sister, who has end-stage chronic obstructive pulmonary disease (COPD), is rapidly deteriorating. The patient had requested to die at home and the district nurses had been visiting twice a day to manage her palliative care and support the family.

The patient is having respiratory difficulty and, despite the oxygen, is increasingly distressed. Written up for analgesia, analytics and sedation, her agitation is frightening for the family and they are asking if they should call the ambulance. The team leader initially says yes but Ruth speaks up and says she will go and assess.

(Continued)

(Continued)

The team leader puts down the phone and challenges Ruth that the family may make a complaint that the care was not handled well and that Ruth may get tied up for the rest of the afternoon with the situation, but Ruth stands her ground and goes. On arrival she finds the patient in distress and the family upset. She explains what is happening and repeats previous discussions about what to expect at end of life. Talking calmly to the patient who is not fully conscious she administers medication and sits with the family until the patient settles. Once the patient is calm she listens to the worry of the family and explores the wishes of the patient to stay at home. She acknowledges the distress this causes the family and asks them gently what they want. They agree they want her to stay with them at home and feel less anxious about what has just happened and if it happens again. Ruth reassures them she is on until the end of the day and that she will give a full handover to the night staff who will come if needed. Two hours later Ruth gets a call to say she has died peacefully and the family are waiting for the GP to come and certify their loved one's death.

Reflections on Ruth's story: Ruth (although she would strongly refute it) displays courage on a number of levels, recognising the culture of avoiding risk to do what she believes meets the needs of her patient. It is her experience, as well as her commitment to stay focused on what the patient wanted, that enabled her to draw the strength to challenge her manager and hold her position.

Courage to enjoy being emotionally involved

In an increasingly pressurised environment and research looking at the emotional labour of caring, it can easily be assumed that caring is synonymous with emotional labour and distress (Hirschhorn, 1988; Menzies Lyth, 1988; Ballatt and Campling, 2011). Yet many will report about the joy of caring and how it gives meaning and purpose to people's working lives. The concept of vocation (from the Latin meaning a 'call' or 'summons') has become less attractive as it can be seen to diminish the professional role that is undertaken by health staff and yet it is often the initial pull for people to pursue a career in this area. Whilst an interest in the sciences (biological and social) is often an underlying drive to apply to work in the environment of healthcare, we would suggest that it is the positive relational aspects of the work and the vocational pull that enable people to stay and ultimately gain meaning from their work. Being able to admit this in a culture of professionalism can be a challenge and many health professionals struggle with this balance.

The British Psychological Society has been exploring this issue with their members in terms of psychologists sharing their own experience of psychological distress and mental health following a letter in the professional journal, *The Psychologist* in 2016. There have been strong views on both sides of the debate with a general view that whilst doing so demonstrates a level of moral courage of the individual professional, there is no evidence that this makes them a more or less effective practitioner.

We see similar debates in the work of the medical profession and challenges about health professionals sharing their own experiences of ill health. What is interesting to observe is that it appears to be more acceptable for medical colleagues to talk about their physical than their mental illness and questions are more likely to be raised about their ability to practise with a mental health illness. A recent tragic case that illustrates this point is the reporting of Dr Wendy Potts, GP, who blogged about her own mental health and subsequently had a complaint made by a patient registered at the surgery, questioning her fitness to practise. She was suspended and an investigation undertaken. She was subsequently found hanging by her partner at her home.

Looking at research into the 'healing relationship' indicates that 'empathic attunement' is key to positive outcomes, this being particularly relevant within the psychologically based illnesses. Empathy was defined originally by Carl Rogers (1959) as: 'To sense the client's private world as if it were your own but without ever losing the "as if" quality'. The opposite perhaps is disregard, where, for example, experiences of mental ill health may be seen as invalid and judged with a withdrawal of love that embodies an acute sense of socialisolation. These feelings link to physio-logical reactions in the hypothalamic–pituitary–adrenal axis with high levels of cortisol production and the associated biological impact of this. This emphasises the importance of authentic empathy, as experienced by patients, and the emotional courage of professionals to sit with the client in a non-judgemental way, even if what they hear or experience is emotionally distressing.

Zender and Olshansky (2012) outline the significance of the 'courage to be' emotionally available as a fundamental construct of caring, that lies in the qualities of intra- and interpersonal relationships. The ability of professionals to provide effective interventions requires an understanding of relational dynamics and the ability to build effective relationships with those in receipt of their care. By deconstructing the dynamic process of face-to-face engagement from a psychobiological standpoint, we can attempt to understand the physiological, emotional, cognitive and behavioural impacts of relational interactions and apply this to the impact of the patient–provider relationship, arguing that high quality relationships lead to high quality health outcomes (see Figure 2.1).

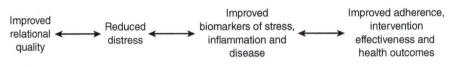

Figure 2.1   Biology of caring

Source: Adapted from Zender and Olshansky (2012)

This understanding is at the heart of care and is one that helps reinforce the case that 'care' is not just a 'nice thing to do', but is key to effective and efficient services. It is therefore critical that health professionals play their role in creating a relationship in which the patient feels a sense of psychological safety and that those managing, commissioning or setting policy for services understand the implications of their actions on this patient–professional interface.

This is particularly important in the context of an ever-increasing commodification of healthcare, which is increasingly being interpreted as a series of tasks, which underplays the significance (and time required) of relationships.

Understanding this allows the patient and the provider to explore what may be helping or hindering building effective relationships and to work together to improve these. It is interesting to note the recent work in introducing health coaches into primary care who have longer appointment times and pay a lot of attention to building effective relationships. This requires the courage to engage in these discussions, both from the patient and the provider perspective, and be able to express shared vulnerability of not only the patient's health but also the skill and effectiveness of the provider in their relational skills.

When courage is observed

In exploring what courage is in practice, Hawkins and Morse (2014) argue that courage had been seen as core to being a nurse from the earlier representation of nurses by people such as Florence Nightingale, but that this definition had diminished over recent years, being replaced by a dominant characterisation of 'caring', in part perhaps due to very public displays of poor care such as the Mid Staffordshire Hospital and Winterbourne View scandals. They suggest that courage in healthcare has several components:

Antecedents – Courage follows a real or perceived threat (to themselves or others), leading to a feeling of vulnerability.

Attributes – Courage manifests itself as a form of advocacy on behalf of the patient and actions (such as taking a stand) despite being fearful of being punished.

Outcomes – As a result of courage, action is taken in the belief they are acting in the best interest of patients.

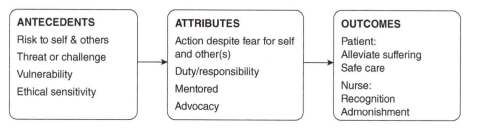

Figure 2.2   Antecedents, attributes and outcomes

Source: Adapted from Hawkins and Morse (2014)

Example from Practice 2.5

Lisa, final-year student nurse

Lisa was a final-year student nurse working on a surgical ward looking after a patient who had developed a secondary postoperative wound infection. The operating surgeon, who had a reputation of having high numbers of postoperative infections, was insisting on a treatment regime, which the nurses disagreed with. Despite trying to discuss this with the surgeon by producing literature reviews on wound management and involving the Tissue Viability Nurses (TVN), the surgeon insisted on his prescription and the wound continued to break down. After a difficult ward round, the surgeon arranged to transfer the patient to another ward. Lisa was transferring at the same time to the new ward and so admitted the patient and continued to treat the wound with the plan advised by the TVN without letting the consultant know. One week post-treatment, the consultant was running the ward round and asked to see the wound, which was now healing well. On examination he was pleased with the results and turned to his team saying that he had moved the patient, as he was concerned about the care from the previous ward. He asked Lisa if she had been looking after the patient, which she confirmed, and asked her how she had been managing the wound. Lisa was torn, as she knew she had not followed his instructions but that the wound was now healing well which the surgeon had openly said to his team. She knew that on behalf of the patient she had done the right thing but now needed courage to stand up for her nursing colleagues and their expertise so described the care plan. The consultant on hearing the intervention used said nothing and moved on, later complaining to the ward manager. Lisa was reprimanded by the manager for embarrassing the consultant but also congratulated on putting the patient's needs first and using the evidence base to deliver care.

Reflections on Lisa's story: Courage can affect change, increase ethical sensitivity and self-actualisation and mitigate moral distress. Lisa learnt the importance of being driven by what was in the patient's best interests, backed up by evidence and the expertise of colleagues and her own ability to stand up for what she believed was the right thing to do.

Courage needs to take place in the context of having some boundaries (Hawkins and Morse, 2014). What we see in practice is when people are unable to be courageous or perhaps their desire to be fails to understand the wider context and as such becomes aggressive or arrogant; it can then lead to becoming distressed and potentially harmful to patient care.

Example from Practice 2.6

Jackie, Learning Set Facilitator

Jackie was running learning sets for senior nursing staff in an acute hospital. A confidential forum, one of the team presented an ethical dilemma she was facing about a disagreement with the general manager who was juggling patients on a waiting list to meet a national target. Whilst the nurse understood the importance of meeting the target, her concern was that patients were sitting on the waiting list having been deemed as low risk without proper screening and that recently there had been several cases come to light that showed patients, not deemed as priority, had been confirmed with cancer. She felt the existing process was placing patients at risk and was experiencing increased distress and anxiety not only about the patients, but also about her role within this.

Having raised this with the manager she had been told that there was no option and that the CEO had been explicit that this was required. The group knew the CEO had a clinical background and were both angry and anxious about the situation and how to deal with it. Jackie knew the CEO from a previous organisation and was convinced that if he knew the details of the situation, he would be concerned and want things reviewed. The initial group response was one of external whistleblowing anonymously as the only option, Working with the nurse and the rest of the group Jackie got her to explore a range of options including gathering data and making an appointment to meet the CEO to discuss concerns and possible options that could remove the risk to patients whilst also meeting the waiting list target. With the support of the group that that would be a sensible first action the nurse gathered her data and went to see the CEO. At the next set the nurse reported that the CEO was indeed extremely concerned about what he was told, thanked the nurse and asked the manager to work together with the nurse to change the process, with a follow-up meeting booked to ensure things were altered. The moral distress she was experiencing prior to the action disappeared and gave her the courage to not only listen to her own judgement but to seek support and advice future situations.

Reflections on Jackie's story: We see here that Jackie helped the nurses explore the boundaries and assumptions held by the nurse about what the CEO wanted and the initial acceptance of the manager's interpretation of the CEO's request. This helped the nurse to not only be courageous but also to manage her moral distress. We explore this further in Chapter 6.

The absence of discussion or education and training around courage in the health professional's curriculum leaves a vacuum in a core concept of providing safe care and is perhaps another consequence of seeing healthcare either as a vocation or simply a profession. These two different frames of reference underplay the emotional elements of care or the energy and courage required to fully connect with the work.

In researching the literature on courage in healthcare, we found it is to be relatively limited and when covered it tends to be found mostly in the nursing literature, yet we would argue its presence, and the need for it, is across all staff working in health and social care, and that it needs to also be addressed at a wider systemic level. With current changes around health and social care and many difficult decisions being made about what is provided, it is essential for those more distant from the actual provision of care to have the courage to connect with what their decisions will mean for those receiving services and those providing it. This is often described as being able to be emotionally detached to make rational decisions. We would argue that if you are really to do the work of healthcare this emotional detachment is counterproductive and that policy makers and senior leaders have to have the courage to engage emotionally as well as logically with this work.

It is interesting to note that what enables courage is often an ethical response to situations in which patients are perceived to be at risk. For staff providing direct care, the risks are visible and often visceral – the greater the distance from the patient the harder it is to experience the risk at a visceral level. This may explain why those health professionals who are in senior positions and no longer in practice do not always recognise the risk and feel the fear of harm to the patient, which acts as the catalyst for action. One of the criticisms that is often levied at senior nurses is that they leave clinical practice relatively early in their career compared to medical colleagues, which could contribute to their perceived inaction against speaking out on safe staffing and patients facing staff's anxiety on risk. This criticism is also levied at managers without a clinical background who have not experienced the emotional aspects of providing care at the patient–practitioner interface.

Whilst not subscribing to the view that a clinical background is essential for those in management, an ability to connect emotionally with the experience of staff and patients is.

Hawkins and Morse (2014) found courage present in ethical–moral 'risk-taking' action(s) despite fear for self and others with the intent to ensure safe patient care. They define four core attributes, which can enhance the presence of courageous acts, as:

- Risk-taking action despite fear for self and other(s) expended directly or indirectly to ensure patient safety
- Duty and responsibility reinforced both internally and externally

- Learned, practised and with help from mentors
- Manifested in advocacy.

When looking at the implications for nursing and safety, Hawkins and Morse (2014) recognise the connection that often occurs between the need for courage and instantaneous action, which can reduce the opportunity for reflection on consequences of action which may lead to problems compromising safety and quality. For example, staff may intervene from their own perspective (own moral code/belief) or not have all the facts at their disposal. This was recently demonstrated in the case of a nurse in a care home who did not carry out cardiopulmonary resuscitation (CPR) on a resident who had died but had no medically signed order to not resuscitate (Spearpoint, 2017). Hawkins and Morse argue that because courage initiates action it is critical for patient safety.

Courage often comes from the combining of one's personal and professional attributes. Having experienced similar experiences to those of patients, professionals who may not have spoken up before against practices seem to find a stronger voice to do so. You see this in the reference above when staff become patients. This is often influenced by personal and professional life experiences of vulnerability and suffering which act either as an eye-opener to others' suffering or a blind spot; courage appears as a significant unifying phenomenon which manifests itself in enabling courage to help patients face their own vulnerability and suffering, and courage to trust oneself in arguing for and providing professional care (Thorup et al., 2012).

The ability of health professionals to process and handle their own feelings is an important factor in being able to handle a patient's feelings related to their vulnerability and suffering. It takes courage to confront patients with their own vulnerability and suffering, particularly when patients may be denying the need for assistance or not facing their vulnerability. Staff enter into the patient–professional relationship without knowing what will happen, and being willing to bear witness and be available both physically and emotionally for what arises is difficult. Far too often, space to process this emotional work is not available or is seen as unnecessary.

Example from Practice 2.7

Jenny, specialist nurse

Jenny was a specialist nurse who believed that care for people with dementia in the hospital was not good enough and looked at ways of continuously improving. Her work for patients resulted in training staff in increased awareness and ways to interact effectively with people with dementia. Whilst improving other people's experience, Jenny also had to deal with her own mother's dementia, which, whilst extremely difficult, also gave her the courage to continually advocate for other.

In addition, it can take time, experience and persistence to trust one's own view and argue for and provide professional care.

Example from Practice 2.8

Kerry, matron

Kerry was the matron for older people in an acute hospital who felt that the environment in which care took place was not conducive to effective rehabilitation. The day rooms had been removed from wards and so there was nowhere to provide any social and physical activity for patients other than individually by their bed which she believed delayed their progress. Her continued raising of the issue, working with a charity and galvanising support led eventually to money being raised and day rooms reinstated and subsequently held up as an essential resource for older people facilitating their rehabilitation and earlier discharge.

It can also be difficult to challenge one's own professional group on points of ethics, such as decreased standards of care:

Example from Practice 2.9

Esther, lead nurse

Esther was the lead nurse for paediatrics and was having difficulty working with the manager of the ED department who saw her as obstructive to plans for redesigning the paediatric area and was pushing for her to be moved. An external consultant was brought in to support the project and went to meet with Esther to understand what the issues were from her perspective. Esther highlighted a number of risks that she perceived with the new configuration. After several minutes of listening to the concerns, the consultant became aware of a feeling of anxiety and distress and reflected that back to Esther, asking if the risks she was describing had ever happened to her. Esther paused and then became tearful as she described the death of a child which she believed was due to the layout of the unit she had been working in. The consultant listened and, when Esther had finished, thanked her for sharing the story. She then asked Esther if there were any other factors that had influenced that situation and what else she believed needed to be in place to prevent this issue. As Esther unpicked the situation she could see that the layout was

(Continued)

(Continued)

one of many factors but that she had attributed everything to this and the discussion around the unit had resurfaced these emotions. It was Esther's very difficult personal experience, her present level of authority and strong desire to protect children that was sustaining her in the difficult interactions she had been having with the manager.

Reflections on Esther's story: It took courage for Esther to get back in touch with the difficult experience but also to be resolute in her challenge to what she felt would risk patient care. Being an experienced and established senior nurse gave her the courage to stand up and say that this was not acceptable.

Often earlier experiences where we have perhaps not spoken up but seen the consequences can motivate us to not repeat the pattern.

The importance of experience

This ability to draw on experiences as a way of strengthening ethical and moral courage is important. Ethical formation as a result of personal attributes and professional qualifications can be seen as a process which occurs over time, which raises the issue of how to keep experienced health professionals directly delivering and supervising care. All too often, for non-medical staff to progress either through expanding their knowledge or their income they need to move into managerial positions or away from direct patient care, which dilutes the expertise at the point of care. It is at this point that the emotional work happens and where the greatest risk of error is present and a lack of knowledge or courage to speak up is a safety concern.

Courage is an integral part of clinical practice. By making it a visible phenomenon that needs to be actively encouraged and supported, it will effectively contribute to an improved health service. The practice of registered nurses working at an advanced level in a variety of clinical settings found that courage is a context-specific, yet universal phenomenon which compromises of numerous interdependent and simultaneously interacting components or parts, and paradoxically is both visible and invisible (Spence and Smythe, 2007). The value of postgraduate education is more than imparting knowledge – it is also to encourage and nurture curiosity, critical thinking and develop confidence, providing strategies to enable staff to stand up and say something effectively. This is a core role of clinical educators as 'critical resistors' to ensure the classroom is a place where the status quo can be challenged (McEldowney, 2003). Education can certainly foster the development of courage. As discussed earlier, one of the authors' own nurse training was underpinned by a consistent message of the role of advocate for patients who were unable to advocate for themselves. This responsibility, expectation and associated authority from the lecturers, would give courage to clinical staff to speak out and question decisions when patients, who often confide in students or more junior staff (who would be spending the majority of their time directly with them, share their anxieties or concerns about treatment plans. It is interesting to reflect whether there is something in the dynamic of this relationship that enables a patient's vulnerability to be sensed, and then heard by more junior staff. Perhaps the presence of the patient's anxiety is mirrored in the junior staff's own anxiety and thus recognised more easily?

Example from Practice 2.10

Jane, registered community nurse

Jane was a community registered nurse who had been asked to visit a woman in her 80s by the GP for a dressing following a fall. The woman lived alone with no close family input or carers. She had been concerned about the woman's cognitive functioning (there was no formal diagnosis of any mental health or neurological condition and no obvious signs of infection) and wanted to monitor it over a few visits. The house was chaotic and Jane would often arrive to find half-eaten plates of food, boxes of medication and the woman unable to recall what she had been doing earlier or sustain a conversation. Whilst the woman had a dossit box for medication, she also had other medication which was prescribed but didn't appear to be taking as directed, including anticoagulants. After a couple of visits Jane persuaded the woman to let her discuss her concerns with the GP and request a visit. Speaking to the GP whilst in the patient's home, Jane encountered resistance with the GP saying she had assessed her several weeks ago and didn't have any concerns so did not feel a home visit was necessary. Jane described the home situation and her concern regarding the woman's cognitive functioning as well as the medication. The GP repeated that she wasn't concerned and that she had a dossit box which the woman was managing. Despite feeling dismissed Jane persevered, saying that she wasn't sure the woman was taking the medication not in the dossit box, in particular her anticoagulant, and wondered when she last had her International Normalized Ratio (INR) checked. The GP tutted and said she would check. After a few minutes holding the GP came back on the line and asked for bloods to be taken. When Jane asked what bloods she wanted and for what purpose the GP admitted that there had been an oversight and that the last INR check had been missed. She then said she would visit the woman the next day.

Clinical supervision can also provide, to some extent, similar support to staff in the practice environment and at the organisational level, as staff need to establish effective ways of working collectively to strengthen all members of the team's voice in multidisciplinary forums (Spence and Smythe, 2007).

The role of a clinical tutor is extremely important but, in reality, heavy caseloads can mean staff are not always able to support the students or junior staff. A clinical tutor provides a dedicated and slightly more objective support structure that can model challenge to others as a way of teaching students and more junior staff to raise concerns using evidence and experience.

With the recent reduction in mature students entering the nursing profession due to cuts in the bursary, the introduction of nursing associates and physicians assistants as less qualified staff, and a culture where speaking up is not universally welcomed or expected, we would argue that the need for courage has never been greater. In the dynamic of increasingly complex healthcare, the knowledge required is greater and thus there is a risk that these staff will not have that knowledge which may make them less confident to speak out when they have concerns. There is also a risk that they are not listened to by those in a hierarchal position, who dismiss their concerns if they are not able to cite the evidence that a degree-educated nurse, advanced practitioner or consultant would have been exposed to.

By having both the experience and the research evidence around what contributes to creating a therapeutic relationship, staff can call for organisational practices that support this. Institutional barriers to good clinical practice, such as organisational commitment to efficiency and the hierarchy of organisational objectives, can result in the marginalisation of 'care', making staff feel less supported in their practice. In an environment that places primacy on efficiency and reducing waste, it risks creating a hierarchy that privileges the biomedical model of disease and cure, discounting the importance of the 'caring' relationship with the patient and family. It also places pressure on the building of relationships with team members as less important than handing patients over to each other to move on to the next patient, creating more task-based and fragmented care.

Working in this context places clinicians' relational role in conflict with the environment they are working in, such that if they take longer to complete a task (e.g. home visit for a 'routine' dressing but the patient is highly anxious or distressed) they may face criticism for delaying the next visit, or asking a physician to explain the rationale for their treatment plan may be met with criticism as to why they need to explain their decision to the pharmacist or nurse, for example.

Single-minded pursuit of outcomes, without consideration of what nurses and patients are forced to become in the process, undermines the essential good in nursing and medicine. Optimal conditions for healing and care within the family system are possible only when nurses, patients and family members are treated as persons and not as commodities to be managed rapidly and inexpensively as possible. The moral ecology of nursing is sustained by institutional structures that allow adequate time for nurses' relational work with patients, families, and colleagues in order to skilfully assess the patients' safety, physiological and emotional needs and to intervene with appropriate timing and care. (Weiss et al., 2002: 107)

In an ever-increasingly financially challenged health system, the ability to resist the push for speed and cost over time and value, becomes difficult and requires not only the courage to challenge, but also the ability to present the case in a format that recognises the reality of the constraints in which the system is operating.

Knowledge and the intuitive understanding inherent in clinical expertise is not enough; courage requires having or finding the necessary energy and being able to endure the stresses to persevere over time. The case study above shows how Jane had to persevere even in the face of being dismissed, to push for her concerns to be taken seriously and acted upon. It can take courage to keep believing in oneself when others do not share that belief and to hold onto your own wisdom that comes from years of experience and deep knowledge, but there is a cost to this which can be psychologically exhausting – being courageous is not easy.

Courage can also be a paradoxical interplay of opposites where it manifests itself both in knowing and unknowing and the simultaneous experiencing of fear and confidence. When faced with decisions, you may only really know the correctness of your decision after the event. We see this in the case of Steve in Chapter 3.

What we see throughout the chapter and this book is that context can, both in terms of 'other' and organisational and systemic structures, support or hinder courage. It can take considerable courage for health and social care staff professionals to be visible and to communicate clearly and forcefully in a service which they see as dominated by technical rationalist discourse (Polkinghorne, 2004). It takes courage to assert and practise healthcare as a caring and moral endeavour. It can also take courage to keep going and stay in touch with the developments in research and national policy which influence the delivery of healthcare. Sometimes after a difficult shift it can even take courage to come back the next day.

Finally, we see in this chapter and in Chapter 4, the significant physical and emotional impact of illness and death on those experiencing it and those who care for them (be they health and social care professionals or friends and family). This sits at the core of the patient–professional relationship and requires the courage of all involved to recognise the emotional work and courage of the other. It is in this understanding of the 'other' that the conditions required for 'courageous care' are created together.

Useful Weblinks

www.nuffieldtrust.org.uk/media/jonathon-tomlinson-at-summit-2018-reflections-on-the-welfare-state-from-primary-care

Valerie Iles shares a moving piece on the experience of her mother's death: www.reallylearning.com/dying-is-the-most-grown-up-thing-we-ever-do-so-lets-take-it-seriously

www.rcot.co.uk/sites/default/files/COT-Professional-Standards_0.pdf

www.pointofcarefoundation.org.uk/our-work/schwartz-rounds

www.pulsetoday.co.uk/home/finance-and-practice-life-news/bipolar-gp-dies-by-suicide-following-patient-complaint-about-online-blog/20032669.article

https://counsellingresource.com/features/2007/10/09/empathy-as-if

References

Aiken, L.H., Clarke, S.P., Sloane, D.M., Sochalski, J. and Silber, J.H. (2002) 'Hospital nurse staffing and patient mortality, nurse burnout, and job satisfaction', *JAMA, 288*(16): 1987–1993.

Alpers, R.R., Jarrell, K. and Wotring, R. (2012) 'Teaching courage: An essential for nursing education', *Teaching and Learning in Nursing, 7*(3): 121–122.

Ballatt, J. and Campling, P. (2011) *Intelligent Kindness – Reforming the Culture of Healthcare.* London: Royal College of Psychiatrists Publications.

Berne, E. (1964) *Games People Play.* Harmondsworth: Penguin.

Dartington, T. (2010) *Managing Vulnerability: The Underlying Dynamics of Systems of Care.* London: Karnac Books.

Day, L. (2007) 'Courage as a virtue necessary to good nursing practice', *American Journal of Critical Care, 16*(6): 613–616.

Department of Health and Social Care (2010) *Nothing Ventured, Nothing Gained: Risk Guidance for People with Dementia.* Available at: https://assets.publishing.service.gov.uk/government/uploads/system/uploads/attachment_data/file/215960/dh_121493.pdf (accessed July 2018).

Gerrard, N. and Jones, J. (2014) *John's Campaign.* Available at: http://johnscampaign.org.uk/# (accessed 30 May 2018).

Hawkins, S.F. and Morse, J. (2014) 'The praxis of courage as a foundation for care', *Journal of Nursing Scholarship, 46*(4): 263–270.

Hirschhorn, L. (1988) *The Workplace Within: Psychodynamics of Organizational Life.* Cambridge, MA: MIT Press.

Iles, V. (2005) *Managing Change in the NHS* (2nd edn.). Maidenhead: Open University Press.

Iles, V. (2016) 'Dying is the most grown up thing we ever do – so let's take it seriously', *Health Care Analysis, 24*(2): 105–118. Available at: www.reallylearning.com/dying-is-the-most-grown-up-thing-we-ever-do-so-lets-take-it-seriously/ (accessed 30 May 2018).

Kerfoot, K. (1999) The culture of courage, *Nursing Economics, 17*(4): 238–239.

Klitzman, R. (2007) *When Doctors Become Patients.* Oxford: Oxford University Press.

Maben, J., Peccei, R., Adams, M., Robert, G., Richardson, A., Murrells, T. and Morrow, E. (2012) 'Exploring the relationship between patients' experiences of care and the influence of staff motivation, affect and wellbeing', final report, NIHR Service Delivery and Organisation programme.

Maxfield, D., Grenny, J., McMillan, R., Patterson, K. and Switzler, A. (2005) *Silence Kills: Seven Crucial Conversations for Healthcare.* American Association of Critical Care Nurses. Available at: www.aacn.org/nursing-excellence/healthy-work-environments/~/media/aacn-website/nursing-excellence/healthy-work-environment/silencekills.pdf?la=en (accessed 30 May 2018).

McPherson, S., Hiskey, S. and Alderson, Z. (2016) 'Distress in working on dementia wards – A threat to compassionate care: A grounded theory study', *International Journal of Nursing Studies, 53*: 95–104.

McEldowney, R. (2003) 'Critical resistance pathways: Overcoming oppression in nursing education', in N. Diekelmann (ed.), *Teaching Practitioners of Care: New Pedagogies for the Health Professions.* Madison, WI: University of Winsconsin Press. pp. 194–231.

Menzies Lyth, I. (1988) *Containing Anxiety in Institutions.* London: Free Association Books.

Meyer, E. (2014) 'Courage, brains and heart: Lessons from The Wizard of Oz for difficult healthcare conversations', *Australian Critical Care, 27*(3): 108–109.

Nuffield Trust (2018) *Jonathon Tomlinson at Summit 2018: Reflections on the Welfare State from Primary Care*. Available at: www.nuffieldtrust.org.uk/media/jonathon-tomlinson-at-summit-2018-reflections-on-the-welfare-state-from-primary-care (accessed 30 May 2018).

Osterland, J., Ternestedt, B.M, Hansebo, G. and Hellstrom, I. (2016) 'Feeling lonely in an unfamiliar place: Older people's experiences of life close to death in a nursing home', *International Journal of Older People's Nursing*, 12(1).

Peck, S. (1990) *The Road Less Travelled*. London: Arrow.

Point of Care Foundation (n.d.a) *Sweeney Programme*. Available at: www.pointofcarefoun dation.org.uk/our-work/sweeney-programme (accessed 30 May 2018).

Point of Care Foundation (n.d.b) *Schwartz Rounds*. Available at: www.pointofcarefounda tion.org.uk/our-work/schwartz-rounds (accessed 30 May 2018).

Polkinghorne, D. (2004) *Practice and the Human Sciences: The Case for a Judgment-Based Practice of Care*. Albany, NY: State University of New York Press.

Professional Standards of Occupational Therapy Practice (2017) College of Occupational Therapists (p. xi).

Psychologist, The (2016) 'Clinicians with mental health difficulties', 29.

Rogers, C. (1959) A theory of therapy, personaility, and interpersonal relationships as developed in the client-centered framework. In S. Koch (Ed.) Psychology: A study of science, (*Vol.3*, Formulations of the person and the social context). New York: McGraw Hill.

Rodney, V. (2000) 'Nurse stress associated with aggression in people with dementia: Its relationship to hardiness, cognitive appraisal and coping', *Journal of Advanced Nursing*, 31(1): 172–180.

Shapiro, J. (2008) 'Walking a mile in their patient's shoes: Empathy and othering in medical students' education', *Philosophy, Ethics and Humanities in Medicine*, 3(1): 10.

Smith, S.J. (1995) 'The vital link', *Nursing Times*, 91: 51–52.

Spearpoint, K. (2017) 'The implications of NMC caution for nurse who did not perform CPR', *Nursing Times*, 113(7): 18–20.

Spence, D. and Smythe, L. (2007) 'Courage as an integral to advancing nursing practice', *Nursing Praxis in New Zealand*, 23(2): 43–55.

Thorup, C.B., Rundqvist, E., Roberts, C. and Delmar, C. (2012) 'Care as a matter of courage: Vulnerability, suffering and ethical formation in nursing care', *Scandinavian Journal of Caring Sciences*, 26: 427–435.

Weiss, S.M., Malone, R.E., Merighi, J.R. and Benner, P. (2002) 'Economism, efficiency, and the moral ecology of good nursing practice', *Canadian Journal of Nursing Research*, 34(2): 95–119.

Zender, R. and Olshansky, E. (2012) 'Biology of caring; Researching the healing effects of stress response through relational engagement', *Biological Research for Nursing*, 14(4): 419–430.

3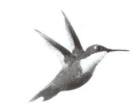

COURAGE TO LEAD

REBECCA MYERS

Courage is not the absence of fear but rather the judgment that something is more important than fear; the brave may not live forever, but the cautious do not live at all. From now on you'll be travelling the road between who you think you are and who you can be. The key is to allow yourself to make the journey.

Meg Cabot

By the nature of the work, healthcare requires difficult decisions to be made. Stepping forward to lead in any scenario, whether as the domestic on the ward to offer a suggestion on how to do something different, to the decision of a politician to invest in some services at the expense of others, can be difficult. When these decisions are filled with difficult emotions, such as fear of getting it wrong, distress at the impact it will have, or upset, leading requires courage.

As part of the response to the emerging findings of the public inquiry into care at Mid Staffordshire Hospital (2013) the Chief Nurse for NHS England developed the 6Cs framework, which indicated that courage is a critical aspect of working in healthcare. But much older lessons can be drawn from the leadership styles of people who have exhibited great courage and brought about change, such as Gandhi or Martin Luther King. But we would suggest that courage to lead isn't just seen as the stereotypical charismatic variety, but also as the daily interactions between staff and patients in achieving good healthcare.

Attempts to 'measure' courage have been limited due to its complexity to describe and discern, but events, such as the Mid Staffordshire Inquiry or the response on 11 September 2011 in New York, has led organisational psychologists (Kilmann et al., 2011) to develop measurement tools to explore the dominant cultures of organisations and how behaviours defined as 'courageous' are exhibited and responded to. Courage and other attributes are needed to overcome resistance to change, to stand strong in the face of criticism or personal attack, and require a targeted sensing of the environment by managers and leaders. This chapter will consider the courage needed by leaders in these everyday operational situations as well as the more extreme situations which can accompany high-profile issues in healthcare.

Caring as leaders

In relation to the 'courage to care' (Chapter 2), caring is not the sole responsibility of health professionals but also of those managing and leading. Valerie Iles (2005) defines 'caring management as it manifests in acts of work and courage that enable the flourishing of patients, staff and colleagues and their own ability to flourish in their service'.

The role of senior leaders in any organisation, be it healthcare or not, is to enable staff to meet the purpose of the organisation. For healthcare its primary task is to care for those at times of ill health and vulnerability, thus the role of the Board (be it individual providers or national bodies) is to create the environment in which care can be delivered. This requires leaders to be courageous in their decisions about performance issues and where to focus resources or how to manage pressures from external influences, be they politicians, regulators or the media. In healthcare, it can be assumed that it is only the clinical staff that require courage and yet staff in corporate departments and facilities are often faced with situations that test their moral courage.

Example from Practice 3.1

Steve, Deputy Director of Finance, District General Hospital

Steve was a Deputy Director of Finance in a large DGH who was becoming increasingly concerned about the financial position and the ask of clinical staff due to the level of vacancies and the volume of activity. He would often be the voice at senior managers' meetings arguing against the reality of budget setting and the need to give nursing staff more flexibility in their recruitment plans to over recruit due to the turnover and the cost of agencies arguing the annual cost of over recruitment would be less than temporary staff costs with their associated profit margins and the wider emotional costs of constant changes in local teams.

His challenge, and increasing concerns about overall control totals, was making him increasingly demoralised and so he and his colleagues would put extra efforts into the charity that he and others had set up to raise money for the hospital. After several years of being vocal not just locally but through various national bodies, he felt the direction of travel financially where he was, was unsustainable and thus spoke publicly

(Continued)

(Continued)

of his concerns and resigned. In an environment that, despite having over 1.5 million staff in the NHS, is still a relatively small organisation, speaking out against the 'system' is not always viewed favourably but he believed his concerns were too great not to and that the personal risk was not as important as the wider implications of not speaking out.

Reflections on Steve's experience: Steve is not alone in the finance world and others have questioned finance decisions on public forums such as Twitter, including public statements by former finance directors on what they believe are unrealistic 'control totals' (overall expenditure levels) which will directly affect the quality and safety of care and staff wellbeing. In 2016, an anonymous letter was sent to the chair of the Public Accounts Committee outlining a series of concerns from an Executive Director, which the Department of Health and NHS England were asked to account for. Whilst anonymous, one should not underestimate the courage required in doing this as unfortunately the risk of being identified and subsequently removed from their position, or career opportunities disappearing, is still not an uncommon response to those who 'speak out' (this features again in Chapter 5 – Courage to Challenge).

All too often, the work of healthcare, which is about providing care both at the individual and population level, creates an inherent tension in how resources are allocated. This tension often gets located in the role of those in managerial positions, many of whom have previously been clinicians themselves. Their motivation to work in healthcare does not shift because they change roles but their areas of responsibility and function do. Having to manage this tension can be emotionally distressing for them and requires them to stay in touch with these emotions to be able to discharge their responsibilities with empathy and effectiveness. Just like the health professional who displays courage in being emotionally available to their patients, those managers who are able to connect with the emotions of their staff who are being asked to deliver, often under extreme service pressures, and patients and families who are often directed to managers when they wish to complain, demonstrate courage in absorbing these emotions and supporting staff at the same time. We shall return to this in Chapter 6.

What is courage in leadership?

Having explored definitions of courage in Chapter 1 we look to explore what this means in the context of leadership.

Courage is part of the structure of organisational life and is occurring on a daily basis from reporting why deadlines are missed to raising a concern about a service or admitting when you have made a mistake (Worline and Quinn, 2003). For those in formal leadership positions there is an added component of visibility, responsibility and therefore accountability as their behaviour is seen as a model of what is expected and in turn greatly influences the culture of an organisation. However, the idea that 'leading' is an omnipotent force that resides in the few has been increasingly challenged (Andrews, 2013) and whilst not wanting to detract from the achievements of those in these formal roles, it is important to consider the wider elements of what is in place when people behave in what might be labelled as 'courageous'.

The analogy of the leader as a *gardener* that can plant the seed, but cannot make it grow unless the conditions are conducive illustrates the importance of context, i.e. the seed and the environment create a self-reinforcing growth process (Senge, 1999). In this framing, leadership is a relational activity and requires those in leadership positions to be able to confront their own behaviours to know when they are contributing to the conditions that stifle growth. This is not always easy and thus we believe it requires them to be courageous.

But courage is also not the monopoly of those in public sector organisations so what makes it different in a healthcare context?

Courage in healthcare leadership

As we explored in Chapter 2, the nature of healthcare is interacting with people at some of the most vulnerable times of their lives. This vulnerability leads to a highly charged emotional context and, coupled with the political context of the work, means that the actions of those within it are subject to higher levels of scrutiny, and the performance of the service is often used for party political purposes. The Secretary of State for Health and Social Care at the time, Jeremy Hunt MP, at the 2015 NHS Confederation Conference on the values of leadership, told the audience that people in the NHS work at the 'intersection between the financial operational and moral aspects of society'.

The NHS has been described as 'the nearest thing to a national religion' (former Chancellor of the Exchequer, Nigel Lawson), which means pressure not only on the Health Secretary and government when they start to govern over changes that are seen as destructive, but also on those managing and working within it. A backdrop of perceptions that those in 'management' positions are driven by different sets of values than those who are providing direct care (Powell and Davies, 2016) means that the motives and value judgements of those in formal leadership positions are often more readily scrutinised and challenged.

It is interesting to explore how healthcare professionals, on seeing the courage displayed by patients and relatives dealing with physical and emotional pain, adjust their own sense of what is courageous and thus are more disarming in their attribution of courage to themselves but also to those in leadership positions. Often unaware of the pressure placed on leaders from the political context, they are unable to see the behaviour other than in the context of their own view of the world.

Psychologists define this as 'attribution theory' (Heider, 1958) where we draw on different data to understand and explain others' behaviours. For clinical staff that are confronted, on a daily basis, with the impact of illness and trauma alongside the consequences of management and policy decisions, it can be difficult to understand the conditions in which these decisions are made or appreciate the courage required at times, leading to a 'fundamental attribution error' (Ross, 1977).

Public acts of courage can serve to raise the moral and social conscience of a society and, due to the link of constructions of moral action, it is often connected to what is 'right' or 'good' as it serves society as a whole (Goldberg and Simon, 1982; Finfgeld, 1999). Thus, the health and wellbeing of all of us when we are vulnerable, and actions that stand up to any violation of that, can be seen as courageous – whistleblowing being a key area which we cover in Chapter 5.

In stories of courageous work performance, strong emotions are interwoven with the 'doing' of the work and the mission of the organisation. In healthcare, when people are seen as standing up for the 'right' thing this is often in: the interests of patients; the wellbeing of staff; investment in research, or against a powerful structure (be that government, regulator or private provider). The emotions evoked when these areas feel under threat, play a mediating role between the need for courage by those in leadership roles and the changed 'sense' of the organisation.

Providers who have been rated as inadequate by the Care Quality Commission (CQC) or placed in Special Measures know only too well how the emotional state of those with influence and power in the organisation can affect the 'sense' of the organisation. When a large teaching hospital was given a provisional rating of 'Requires Improvement', from the CQC, the CEO's open and public challenge of the rating, and the whole regulatory framework, enabled those inside it to maintain an air of confidence and pride in the organisation in the face of a critical review, as opposed to other Trusts who were rated inadequate who described the sense of embarrassment and shame. One of the authors heard from staff who had been publicly criticised and rated poorly:

> When people asked where I worked I didn't say the name of the hospital but the region as I was embarrassed. (Medical consultant)
>
> If I saw people locally who knew I worked at the hospital, I would try and hide as I was ashamed of what the local papers were saying. (Senior nurse)

The response both of the leaders and those powerful players within the 'system' in turn act as a contagion for the whole organisation and will shape the response in the short and long term. It could be argued that when the CEO is seen as powerful and is well connected politically, fighting a rating might be less courageous and more arrogant, especially if there were clear reasons for questioning the quality of services. In this case a more courageous response may have been to publicly accept where there were poor services and to agree a plan for improvement.

The recent CQC critical assessment of a service run by Birmingham Children's Hospital resulted in the CEO tweeting an apology and saying it was not good enough, they had let patients down and were working hard to address the concerns that had been raised. This public acceptance of the review, and commitment to change, signals to the staff, the wider NHS and public that when things are not acceptable an apology is needed and the concerns acknowledged and addressed. Parallels can be drawn here with health professionals who make mistakes and immediately report them and inform the patient and their family of what has happened. Whilst the introduction of a 'Duty of Candour' (first introduced in Chapter 1) through the Health and Social Care Act 2008 has made this a requirement of professionals, an environment that responds in a punitive fashion reduces the likelihood of people reporting these errors. (We will also explore this more in Chapter 6 when we look at the conditions in which courage flourishes.)

Health professionals who do not understand or ignore the political aspects (irrespective of political allegiance) of healthcare deny themselves and their patients the opportunity for improvement. Margaret Hefferman, in her book *Wilful Blindness* (2011), describes how we can prefer ignorance as a way of 'protecting' ourselves from difficult truths or conflict and yet it again requires courage of those in the system to listen to those we disagree with and speak truth to power. Margaret Heffernan argues that the biggest threats and dangers we face are the ones we do not see – not because they're secret or invisible, but because we're wilfully blind. Wilful blindness is a term used in law to describe a situation in which a person seeks to avoid civil or criminal liability for a wrongful act by intentionally keeping himself or herself unaware of facts that would render him or her liable (see https://en.wikipedia.org/wiki/Willful_blindness).

'Wilful blindness', or turning a blind eye deliberately to the point of ignoring deliberate misfeasance, is a disaster in healthcare environments, e.g. the NHS, as it was in 'textbook corporate scandals', such as ENRON. It is highly relevant to the issue of toxic cultures discussed below.

Staying open to the emotional aspects of the work in healthcare and being the 'container' of those emotions for staff who are being asked to deliver 'compassionate' care against a backdrop of high staffing vacancy rates, increased complexity, acuity and volume of patients and rising expectations, means that leaders need to be able to have the emotional courage to 'absorb', process, and be 'emotionally available' to staff experiencing their own emotional responses whilst returning day after day to lead and manage change. People who are able to 'soften the blow' of the emotional pain of others have a high emotional intelligence capacity but, unless they are supported, they run the risk of affecting their own health; thus the courage is required not only to do the work of leading, but also to recognise when you as a leader need help yourself.

Recognising the traditional models of leadership, which were based on the sense of the omnipotent, charismatic, hero leader, contemporary thinking is that leadership is a social 'process' rather than simply the characteristics of individuals. Therefore, it needs to be seen in the context of people's relationships with those that work with and follow them in creating healthy and productive dynamics. In their work looking at effective teams across the NHS, Alimo-Metcalfe et al. (2013) found 'exemplary' leadership operating through the influencing of team activity, ensuring what they found to be three positive outcomes that were critical for high performance: innovation, a focus on quality, and how to continually improve.

In his book, *The Fish Rots from the Head*, Garratt (2010) explores the important role boards play in organisational culture and performance. Boards have two main functions to fulfil: 'conformance' which is dealing with short-term issues and compliance with regulatory conditions and stakeholder accountability; and 'performance' focusing on the longer term perspective to identify the vision and strategy of the organisation. Each of these has an internal and external focus (Searle et al., 2014). In times of pressure such as the current financial position of the provider sector in healthcare and within the political cycle, it is easy for Boards (and external stakeholders such as regulators and politicians) to place increased pressure on the conformance agenda at the expense of the longer term plans and, depending on what is causing the greatest concern, short term cost at the expense of longer term quality. This increased pressure can result in anxiety of Board members and the recognition of the impact of poor behaviour or lack of competence in the boardroom has led to an increase in attention on improving governance and accountability through the concept of a 'unitary board' whereby directors are expected to have an understanding across all portfolios, not simply be there to represent their own positions. This means there is greater expectation and evidence of questioning and challenging information and assumptions across different functions and issues. This way of behaving promotes more of a culture of learning and inquiry through diversity of experience, thinking styles and backgrounds. Information that enables Board members to see quickly what the key issues are and what the board should be focusing on is fundamental.

In addition, a proper induction and annual performance review, including the use of '360 feedback' and board self-assessment tools is important to ensure that a culture of feedback, reflection and learning occurs at the top, creating a learning organisation. Diversity on boards has been a key issue both in terms of gender and ethnic background and a review of characteristics of 'high' performing Trusts identified specifically that Boards that included more female board members and active non-executive directors were associated with better staff and patient experience and higher clinical and financial performance (Chambers et al., 2013). The rationale is that diversity avoids the well-known phenomenon of group think (Janis, 1982), a process whereby groups develop a distinct way of thinking and often fail to adopt a more critical analysis of situations.

Boards need to appreciate how their behavioural styles influence organisations such that there is often an 'amplification affect' whereby leaders' behaviour and comments are assumed to be 'the way to behave' and thus get modelled across the organisation. Demonstrating positive role modelling in terms of listening, dialogue, curiosity and focus on excellence, all signal what leaders value, what gets rewarded and defines a pathway others can follow (Cook and Hoas, 2008).

Example from Practice 3.2

Carol, CEO and former clinician

As a CEO in an organisation under heavy scrutiny for clinical performance, Carol (a former clinician) was faced with a situation where she felt an error of judgement had been made regarding a patient's clinical care prior to her taking up post. The family were pursuing a legal action and Carol had asked to meet with them to hear from them what they felt had happened. Having read the statements from staff, Carol believed that the concerns raised by the family were legitimate and that an alternative course of action could have led to a better outcome for the patient. Although the CEO and thus an authority figure in her own right, Carol was strongly advised by the legal team not to meet with the family on their own or to make any admission of error on behalf of the hospital.

Carol chose to ignore the advice and met with a family representative to discuss what had happened. On hearing the relative's perspective and seeing the on-going emotional distress of the family, Carol not only apologised but also agreed with the family that this may well indicate an error of judgement. Carol recognised the complex and stressful situation in which the staff were working and thus their human fallibility as well as the authority of the legal and clinical team who would not agree with her management of the situation.

This apology and acknowledgment enabled the family to stop blaming themselves and to properly grieve for their loved one.

Carol's subsequent conversation with the clinical team was one of understanding of the context whilst firmly reinforcing the importance of acknowledging when things go wrong. There was no disciplinary procedure but there was training and supervision for the staff involved, to reflect and assure themselves and others that they would manage things differently in the future.

This response sent a clear message to people in the organisation that mistakes happen and they are always distressing but that they need to be acknowledged, apologised for and learnt from.

However, it is not just having a clinical background that guarantees stepping forward. West (2010) in his coverage on the failings of standards of care at Mid Staffordshire, reported that Anthony Sumara, an experienced CEO without a clinical background, when taking over the hospital was clear that there needed to be public acknowledgement of the poor standards of care in order to shift the culture and stated explicitly that staff were expected to speak out against poor practice and that they needed to be listened to (see www.bbc.co.uk/news/uk-england-stoke-staffordshire-11837400).

Families of those affected at Mid Staffordshire pushed leaders and the new CEO to introduce an 'honesty and courage' programme where staff would be shown videos of patients and relatives talking about their experiences with a set of questions for staff to reflect on, including:

- How does that make you feel?
- You are part of this organisation; do you want to say sorry?
- What are you going to do about it in future?

It is important that the request by those in leadership roles for people to step forward and raise concerns, recognises the difficulty those in more junior positions can face. The ability to predict others' responses to situations and the willingness to act may be limited as we may over/under estimate based on our own willingness and ability to act (Van Boven et al., 2005).

This 'over-confidence' about responses in hypothetical situations, presents useful reflections for people who take a stand assuming others will follow, particularly when the perceived emotional impact may be costly. Fear of embarrassment, or worse, is an important determinant of social behaviour and thus being able to accurately predict the fear of embarrassment or other consequences will assist in interpreting social behaviour.

An underestimation of the impact of fear on their own preferences and decisions to act, can lead to an 'illusion of courage' and an 'empathy gap' because people do not anticipate how much emotional arousal influences how they will react.

Insight of those who lead

Sometimes what stops leaders from behaving in a way that is effective and enables others to raise concerns is a lack of feedback or self-awareness of the impact they are having on others. In an honest and difficult reflection, a former CEO, Kate Grimes, shares how hard it was to give her honest feedback and how her style had led to people perceiving her as a bully (see www.hsj.co.uk/workforce/bullying-in-the-nhs--a-bullys-perspective/7020654.article). Whilst it is easy to point the finger and say people in these positions 'should' be self-aware and 'should' be able to manage their emotions, these roles are incredibly pressurised and the dynamic between those who lead and those who report to them is a complex one. There is a responsibility on those around to be able to give constructive feedback to those in senior positions if they see a pattern of behaviour which is destructive to creating an environment that facilitates honesty and the ability to raise concerns.

Much understanding of the inherent risk in healthcare safety is recognised in the work of Martin Bromiley (2007) who founded the Clinical Human Factors Group – a charity set up after the death of his wife following a 'routine' surgical operation (see: www.youtube.com/watch?v=JzlvgtPIof4). A pilot by training, his work with clinical colleagues studies human factors that influence performance and how to counter these to reduce errors or risks to safety. Bromiley's work focuses primarily on the role of human factors in the clinical setting; however the wider context in which clinical care takes place also requires an understanding and mitigating strategies for the fact that those in authority should be seen as having both 'legitimate authority and human frailty'. This requires followers who can 'at times be able to question them, correct them, or even disobey them because we can't just say we were following orders' (Chaleff, 2015).

Courage to call out 'toxic' cultures and leadership

In looking at how leadership affects the ability of courage to flourish, it is important to consider how those in formal positions of authority exercise their influence and power over others. Unfortunately, toxic leadership is still present in much organisational life. The latest NHS Staff Survey showed a high percentage of staff reporting high rates of bullying (see www.nhsstaffsurveys.com/Caches/Files/P3088_ST17_National%20brief ing_v5.0.pdf). The implications of this are discussed later in Chapter 4.

Dysfunctional leadership can be characterised by a distinct set of behaviours which include: denying when you are wrong; defending your view despite evidence to the contrary; demonising others who expose facts that expose you; and trying to destroy the career or reputation of anyone who exposes or threatens you (Ellis, 2014).

Tackling this is crucial as it leads to a toxic and unsafe environment and requires courage on the part of other leaders to tackle this behaviour.

Examples from Practice 3.3

Phillipa, Senior Manager

Philippa was a senior manager who disagreed with an investment decision by a colleague which, whilst beneficial in the short term, she felt placed the organisation at greater risk in the longer term without any real plans to mitigate this risk. The colleague had spoken to other executive members before the meeting to get their support but Philippa's requests to meet and discuss concerns were met with silence. On the day of the meeting their behaviour towards Philippa was aggressive and belittling, with a questioning of the competence of her team on a piece of work in front of the Chair having not raised any concerns previously and for which Philippa had no knowledge of any previous issues with the work.

During the meeting the investment proposal came up for discussion and was presented to the non-executive directors (NEDs) as something that had agreement from the

(Continued)

(Continued)

whole executive team. Philippa could feel her pulse rate rising and the anxiety of speaking up and keeping quiet against the tension of what she believed the role of an executive was and so indicated to the Chair that she had a point to raise. She could sense the annoyance of her colleague and the intensity of his look as she said that whilst she could see the benefits in the short term she had concerns about a longer-term financial risk and thought there needed to be greater assurance on how this would be minimised or mitigated altogether. Before her colleague could respond, one of the NEDs spoke up and said they shared Philippa's concerns and felt that if they negotiated an adjustment to the contract this could minimise this risk. The proposal was agreed subject to the adjustments and the meeting moved on. After the meeting the colleague ignored Philippa but reported to other members of the team that she should stick to her own portfolio and that he would not be supporting any ideas she subsequently brought to the table.

Reflections on Philippa's experience: What gave Philippa the strength to speak up despite her anxiety was a strong belief in:

- Safeguarding public money
- The responsibility she held as an executive director
- Belief in the concept of a unitary board
- A willingness to be wrong but not to be silenced
- Standing up to bullying and intimidation to prevent it continuing.

Philippa had not approached the NED before the meeting, as having spoken to one of the executive colleagues they had said that the director had been working on this proposal for months and any challenge would result in a fury and unpleasantness, which was not worth it, so Philippa should just keep quiet. This illustrated the collusion that was happening in the team and a lack of willingness to confront bad behaviour, with Philippa taking on the role of critic for the group.

In an article entitled 'Changing toxic organisational culture', the author Nikki Walker (n.d.) writes, 'In a positive organisational culture, courageous leaders foster an environment where people can collaborate in the decision-making process to strategically shift culture of the organisation as it becomes more nimble, entrepreneurial, and aligned with positive values.' Followers enable misguided leaders to rise to power and stay there. Her analysis applies psychological principles to Adolf Hitler's Germany and Jeff Skilling's ENRON. Followers are therefore advised to confront the fear and worry of challenging a toxic leader as 'exercising courage' will make you stronger. A good way to repel toxic leadership is to constantly be aware of it developing with regular feedback and ultimately, if repeatedly seen in an individual, to dismiss them, adopting what Robert Sutton (2007) describes as 'The No Asshole Rule'.

Leadership as a relational activity

As we start to see from above, looking at an individual and their actions and categorising it as courageous simplifies a more complex issue. By looking at this as more of a continuum from the individual to a set of complex relationships, be it with others or structures, philosophies or paradigms, we start to get a better understanding of the contributions and interplay of the many different facets.

Martin Buber (1923) argues that human life (and all that it represents) finds its meaningfulness in relationships. Whilst putting to one side the religious leanings of Buber's work, understanding that one cannot truly separate oneself from what is around us (I–thou) even if one chooses to see it as separate from ourselves (I–It) enables us to see the importance of relationships and the attention required to understand them and stay in them in a generative way.

Harbour and Kisfalvi (2014) offer a conceptual framework in which we can understand courage in managerial behaviour as the interplay of the individual and management context (see Figure 3.1).

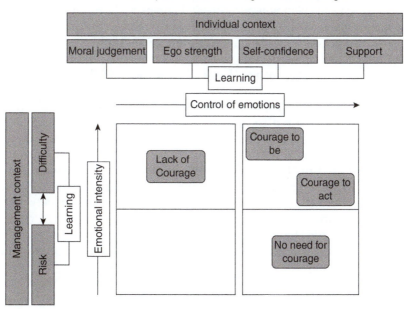

Conceptual model of managerial moral courage

Figure 3.1   Moral courage

Source: Adapted from Harbour and Kisfalvi (2014)

For us in the world of health and social care, this offers a perspective in which we can examine our own and others' behaviour and develop a narrative upon which we can build, to not only teach those in managerial positions, but also to begin conversations about what we would define as morally correct behaviour and how to create the conditions for this to become the norm.

Followership

We know that having our authority challenged is not easy and thus helping those in authority to hear the challenge and recognise its positive intent is important and sits with the point above about personal responsibility and accountability. We need to help people to be 'Courageous Followers' where we are able to build effective relationships with those in authority. A relationship which enables one to speak candidly and act with integrity is essential if you are to be listened to and have your point heard and responded to whilst preserving the relationship, converting 'a hierarchical relationship into a productive partnership' (Chaleff, 2009).

To be able to assume this responsibility followers need to: understand their own power and how to use it; appreciate the values of leaders and their important contribution, playing their role in creating the conditions where leaders' strengths are magnified to serve the common purpose; and understand the seductiveness and pitfalls of the power of leadership which can lead to hubris – 'Power tends to corrupt, and absolute power corrupts absolutely' (Acton, 1837–1869).

Being mindful of these conditions can assist us in not falling into the trap of the parent–child relationship (Berne, 1964), but avoiding an unproductive dynamic that ultimately is a disservice to those involved and the wider purpose of healthcare. One strategy that can assist is getting leaders and followers to be clear about, and connected to, the overall purpose, with their actions always guided by this. Courageous followers should not need to focus solely on meeting the needs of the leader. In health and social care leaders should recruit people who are committed to the purpose of these services and who will remind the leader and others when actions appear to be counter to that. Being a courageous follower is not something that has been explored particularly widely and those who adopt this critical role often go unrecognised in terms of public recognition for their contribution. But these individuals are often able to provide the supportive challenge to leaders in a way that those in whistleblowing situations have not managed to achieve.

Chaleff (2009) offers a framework for followers to consider which enhances the chance of maintaining a partnership relationship and the part the follower has to play in that by the level of challenge and support (see Figure 3.2). Followers who are 'implementers' are high in support and low on challenge, and they can effectively execute the tasks but rarely challenge the norm. Followers who are 'resourcers' are low on support and low on challenge, and only do enough to retain their positions (Chaleff, 2009). Followers who are 'partners' are high on support and high on challenge, and they have more responsibilities. The last type of followers are 'individualists' who are low on support and high on challenge, and their behaviours are more maverick, having fresh ideas but being reluctant to collaborate with others. Rather than seeing these as fixed positions we would suggest people may have developed a pattern for these behaviours which, when reflected back to them, they can modify to be more helpful in achieving organisational purpose.

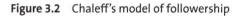

Followership Style

	Low Challenge	High Challenge
High SUPPORT	**IMPLEMENTER** Dependable Supportive Advocate Defender Respectful of authority Reinforces leader's perspective	**PARTNER** Purpose driven Mission orientated Risk taker Cultivates relationship Holds self & others to account Peer relationship with authority
Low SUPPORT	**RESOURCE** Present Available Extra pair of hands Uncommitted Executes minimum requirements Complains to a third party	**INDIVIDUALIST** Confrontational Forthright Self-assured Independent thinker Rebellious Self-marginalising

Figure 3.2 Chaleff's model of followership

Source: Adapted from Chaleff (2009)

Breaking down the component parts of what enables followers to be courageous includes the courage to: assume responsibility – both for yourself and your organisation and its purpose; serve their leader by looking to unburden and support them in the difficult decisions; challenge when they feel discomfort about behaviours or decisions; participate in transformation and champion the need for change when not doing threatens the common purpose; take moral action when needed including against the leader due to a higher set of values; speak to the hierarchy, in a considered and sensitive manner even if not high up in it; listen to others and be open to hearing and adopting different and even opposing views from those who you lead (Chaleff, 2009). Clearly this is not a 'risk-free' list of dimensions due to all the issues we have described around power, politics and emotions, but by becoming more practised and skilful at this way of following it creates more possibility for this to become the norm.

Example from Practice 3.4

Leslie, middle manager

Leslie was a middle manager in a large teaching hospital who had been asked to work with one of the breast surgeons about his high follow-up ratio and the length of his waiting time for new patients. After several attempts to meet him via his secretary and email she decided to wait for him after his clinic. Reluctantly he agreed to see her and made no attempt to hide his irritation at her being asked to get involved. Leslie explained she wasn't there to make any judgements but to help him and the patients who were clearly upset about the waiting time. She asked what the process was for follow-up and he told her he followed all his patients up annually for five years post-treatment and only discharged them if they were disease-free for the five years. This way he felt any recurrence could be picked up quickly and he wasn't prepared to change that. Leslie could see he was extremely committed to his patients and wanted to have a safety net built into their management post-treatment. Leslie reflected that back to him and he agreed, engaging with her a bit more. She asked how many recurrences of cancer were found in these patients at their annual review. The surgeon looked at her for a moment and then said he didn't know. Leslie offered to undertake a study to find out, to which, having been initially reluctant to engage with her, he agreed.

The study revealed that there were a handful of women who had been found to have a recurrence and in all these cases the patient had found a lump several months earlier but, as they had a follow-up, had not presented earlier – thus the 'safety net' had in fact become a risk to starting treatment as soon as possible. On presenting the findings to the consultant he agreed for Leslie to work with him and the team to look at alternative ways of managing the follow-up care, which involved better education of patients post-treatment and a guarantee of direct access to the breast nurse with any concerns. This freed up significant follow-up appointments, improved the experience for patients and utilised the expertise of the multi-disciplinary team and made his outpatient clinic more manageable and pleasant.

Reflections on Leslie's experience: In effect, Leslie had been a courageous follower shifting a hierarchical relationship into a productive partnership.

What actually happens in practice?

As we start to have a better understanding of what is meant by courage, and appreciate the context of leadership in healthcare, we are able to understand the behaviour of those in a leadership situation and the factors that enable them to take these 'courageous' decisions.

Example from Practice 3.5

Kate, CEO, District General Hospital

Kate was a first time CEO of an underperforming district general that had had three different CEOs in the space of five years. A local resident, Kate had both a professional and personal investment in the success of the organisation.

With a severely out-of-date estate and a significant maintenance backlog, Kate knew that the hospital was in much need of capital investment. Introduced by the Conservative Government in 1992, the Private Finance Initiative was the most likely way of raising capital as the Trust had minimal reserves and an inability to borrow money on the open market, as it had not been able to reach Foundation Trust status.

A long-term reconfiguration plan meant that a major service re-development had been thwarted by heavy political interest and, with most of its activity being emergency based, income projections remained moderate.

Requirements for meeting the investment through PFI ran the risk that the Trust would be unable to repay the annual premiums if projections around activity failed to materialise.

The organisation had lived with a poor estate, lack of strategic progress and a poor reputation for many years. Whilst there were pockets of excellent services there were also clinical concerns, some of which were related to the clinical environment the Trust was operating in.

The submission of the PFI bid and signing of the contract with the private partner was not only giving the organisation an option for improvement but also creating longer-term risk to its financial viability.

Kate knew that whilst the repayments based on activity assumptions were possible, due to other interdependent variables the probability of not achieving the activity levels and associated income was high.

Faced with this pressure Kate took the decision to sign the deal against large opposition both locally and nationally around the controversial arrangements of PFI.

Her ability to take the decision – which was seen by some people as a significant career risk if it went wrong – was due to a reliance on her wider network for technical advice as well as her own values and beliefs around the ethical and moral arguments about access to high quality healthcare for a population that often struggled to be heard or represented.

Reflections on Kate's experience: Whilst Kate had a significant power base as the CEO there were still significant personal risks. This case highlights the need for courage when weighing up risk of a financial and strategic nature and having the courage of her belief in implementing a new direction and controversial vision.

But courage as a leader is sometimes about challenging more nebulous issues such as culture.

Example from Practice 3.6

Isabel, Director

Isabel was a first-time director recruited to 'change' the culture of a large healthcare provider. The post had been created after a piece of inquiry about perceptions of a high bullying culture across the organisation.

The organisation had recently completed an extensive financial savings programme and was part of a sector-wide reconfiguration threatening the independent status of the organisation and its provision of services.

As an 'academic' institution, this was their first Director of Organisational Development (OD) alongside a separate Director of Workforce, Mark – someone new to the NHS and also in their first director position. Within the first week the Director of Workforce sent a proposal to the CEO to combine the posts and restructure the whole workforce and OD function.

Isabel had started to make contact with staff across the organisation from different disciplines and levels of the hierarchy and was beginning a series of conversations to understand, 'what was it like to work here?' Early conversations were already identifying themes, which were enabling the perception of 'bullying' to be understood.

Isabel was asked to report to the CEO, shown the report by the Director of Workforce and asked what her plan was. Anxious to be seen as competent and also to do justice to her inquiry and those colleagues who had shared their experiences, Isabel said that whilst she was already gathering 'data' she felt it would be unwise to make any conclusions at this stage and needed to conduct a longer inquiry.

The CEO, who had a reputation for decisive action, agreed reluctantly to give Isabel three more weeks to produce a report.

The on-going inquiry started to identify unhealthy dynamics between the Chair and the CEO with members of the executive team going directly to the Chair and NEDs about issues. Stories played out in the organisation of meetings where staff had felt publicly humiliated for not performing and would then go to meetings and not speak and others who had witnessed this would try to avoid eye contact in case they were targeted. People described having physical symptoms of distress when having to go down the executive corridor with their heart rate increasing as they reached the CEO office.

Occupational health data was indicating high numbers of staff attending for stress and anxiety. Interviews with executive colleagues, the Chair and NEDs repeated the stories played out by staff.

As the end of the month came closer Isabel felt increasingly anxious and con-flicted about what to do. She knew that the purpose of her role and her success criteria were based on the change in the culture. She also knew that a major con-tributory factor was the behaviour of the CEO and the relationship between him and the Chair.

The week that the report was due Isabel asked to meet with the Chair again. She reflected back to the Chair her observations of the CEO/Chair relationship and the impact she saw that having on the CEO, executive team and subsequently the organi-sation. Initially shocked the Chair explored with Isabel their own contribution to the situation and what they needed to consider doing differently if they wanted to trans-form the culture of the organisation.

Isabel was careful not to 'take sides' or make judgement but to stay curious and empathic in the spirit of being helpful. Isabel felt a loyalty to the CEO as a director and at the same time a loyalty to the staff who had been courageous with her in sharing their experiences.

The day before the report was due Isabel sat down with her husband and shared her concerns that if she sent this report she ran the risk of being fired or targeted. She also shared that if she didn't write an honest report she would be doing people a disservice and nothing would change. As the main earner in the household they both knew the risks associated with this and Isabel's husband said he would support her whatever she decided.

The next day Isabel booked a meeting with the CEO for 9am the following day and at 4pm sent the CEO the report marked 'confidential'. Isabel didn't tell anyone what was in the report or that she had sent it. She walked round the organisation chatting to staff, conscious that she may well be asked to leave.

The next morning Isabel went in to see the CEO. Isabel could feel her heart rate increasing but said nothing. The CEO placed Isabel's report down in front of her and said, 'I have read your report'. He looked at Isabel and said; 'You are either extremely naïve or wise, but which ever you are brave'.

Isabel was unsure of what was coming next. Then the CEO said; 'I recognise what you have written; I need you to help me change it'.

Isabel relayed how her respect for the CEO increased significantly. Whilst it was not an easy report to write it was an extremely difficult report to receive and the CEO had taken on board what had been said and took Isabel into his confidence to enable them to change things.

Reflections on Isabel's experience: If we look back at this through the lens outlined above we see the personal resources that Isabel drew upon as well as the wider influences, in particular what she saw as the courageous acts of her colleagues who had shared their experiences and feelings of fear and distress in working in the organisation.

In both Isabel and Kate's situations, we see a number of factors at play that enable them to both 'be' and 'act' courageously (Harbour and Kisfalvi, 2014) as they managed the complex interplay between the facets of organisational life, individuals and situations. In both examples, the situation had moral dimensions, which legitimised organisational interests, and held sway over personal ones and, despite the risky and difficult situation, the outcomes were positive and ethical.

The *courage to act* is the most common type of managerial courage observed and yet the *courage to be* (which is more about dealing with the emotional aspects of situations) is often not appreciated, discussed or visible and is only seen in the most difficult cases (Harbour and Kisfalvi, 2014). The *courage to act* is dealing with a strategic project in a context of conflict or ambiguity, but the person is so convinced of the project's benefits for the organisation that they make a decision and take a position that can either have a positive or negative impact on their career (see the case study of Kate).

The *courage to be* is being able to be in control of your emotions under extreme pressures and the courage to be tenacious and consistent. This is often when the individual is not in control of events. The control of emotions is present and maintained but only with significant effort. The emotional level is experienced as intense because the 'risk' has given way to actual difficulty, requiring great effort to control the emotional response.

Factors that facilitate the manifestation of courage are: the conviction that the work is the right thing to do for the organisation; a high degree of self-confidence; a strong sense of self; expertise and development of skills through past learning; support from the organisation, environment or family and friends; and finally a positive assessment of the consequences of having mobilised the moral courage to act. Acting courageously can be learnt in two ways: through experience or through imitation (Harbour and Kisfalvi, 2014). People who have had to manage risky situations can draw on these experiences at other times when faced with risk, and through observation others can be inspired to confront difficulties and take action. This holds especially true in the clinical context of caring explored in Chapter 2.

However, support from the organisation, the environment or family and friends plays a key role in bolstering self-confidence and moving from courageous decisions to courageous actions.

Reflections on both Kate's and Isabel's experiences: Both Kate and Isabel, having had a positive outcome, had a sense of accomplishment and satisfaction from having acted with integrity, which can bolster self-confidence and act as a motivation to act again if required.

When looking further into courage to act and courage to be, a possible way to reconcile these is to look at courage through a philosophical lens. Here courage is a voluntary act, which emerges from a judgement (courage to act) and through a psychological lens, which suggests courage is an individual's capacity to control their fear (courage to be). This *courage to be* is of particular interest when looking at healthcare where staff feel inferior and at how they can manage this to still express and regulate their emotions in a constructive way to carry out positively deviant (against organisational norms for the greater good) acts. We are seeing more encouragement for staff to engage in this type of behaviour through initiatives such as the School for Health Care Radicals (NHSE Horizons Team) and the Institute for Health Improvement's (IHI) work on 'Breaking the Rules', but this still focuses on an individualistic perspective and needs to be considered in the wider organisational context for actions to be effective and to meet the definition of courage as described above.

Courage to be vulnerable

Chapter 5 explores how people, through being unable to be heard or navigate the organisational context to address concerns, have resorted to 'whistleblowing' through external means. Alongside case studies of people in the 'system' we see examples of courageous leadership from people 'outside'.

Julie Bailey CBE is founder of Cure the NHS, a group she established in December 2007 after the death of her mother at Mid Staffs Foundation Trust Hospital. The group successfully campaigned for a public inquiry into the failings at the hospital and the wider NHS (see www1.bps.org.uk/system/files/user-files/Division%20of%20Clinical%20Psychology/public/cpf263_extended_final.pdf) (Bailey, 2012, 2014).

Tommy Whitelaw, through his mother's experience of care when she had dementia, believes that it only takes one great nurse, care assistant or neighbour to make a difference. And no matter what their role and potential are, their ability to reach out, be respectful and show kindness can have an enormous and positive impact (see: www.dementiauk.org/tommys-story).

Both these individuals (and many others) have different stories and experiences but have stepped forward in the face of significant personal difficulties and sometimes in the face of heavy public criticism to lead the push for change and ultimate improvement in the way healthcare is delivered. This work not only requires significant effort but also courage to continually relive the experiences of their pain and loss in the service of others.

Being in touch with one's own vulnerability can lead to the opportunity to exercise greater strength and courage whilst offering relief and release for others. When we are able to connect with the vulnerability of others, and in turn our own, it can enable us to see our acts in a wider context. Younie (2016) describes how health professionals who share their own sense of vulnerability with students create 'permission' for others to connect to the experiences of patients which in turn offers a different and more compassionate way of relating. It is the ability, individually and collectively, to see vulnerability as an asset, which connects us with others but does not consume us so we become overwhelmed by it, that offers the opportunity to do great work together.

Brené Brown (for example, her TED Talk, available at: www.ted.com/talks/brene_brown_on_vulnerability/transcript?language=en; also Brown, 2015) explores the experience that being comfortable with vulnerability brings, and how this can enable individuals to 'lean' in to difficulties and weather the discomfort. In her research into shame, Brown concluded that feelings of vulnerability were closely aligned to feelings of shame and self-worth.

Those people who could 'sit' with this vulnerability and work through it had a number of things in common:

- Courage – telling your story with your whole heart
- Compassion – self-compassionate as well as to others
- Connection – as a result of authenticity
- Vulnerability – embraced it and believed that their vulnerability was part of who they are and were willing to put themselves out there. We numb vulnerability but we cannot selectively numb as we numb both negative and then positive emotions.
- Changing uncertainty to certainty
- Blame – a way to discharge pain and discomfort

We pretend that what we do doesn't have an effect on people. By letting ourselves be fully seen, our vulnerability diminishes, as there is nothing to hide and it is often the feeling that we need to hide who we really are that keeps us disconnected from others and thus reduces our ability to lead when required. Sharing our vulnerability enables deeper and more meaningful connections with others. The impact of those in 'senior' positions or experienced in their field, sharing their own doubts and mistakes and vulnerability is helpful and inspiring to others, as seen in the work that is carried out in 'Schwartz Center Rounds®', a monthly, confidential forum where staff share their feelings about the work they do through the telling of personal stories. The feedback of the experience of more junior staff who hear leaders talk in this way describes how it helps them to rationalise and process their own emotions and have the courage to speak out or admit when they have made an error or need help.

This sharing of our vulnerabilities is what makes us authentic, as we know that we all have difficulties in different guises and at different times. A denial of that leads to others not experiencing us as genuine, thus leading to an element of distrust.

As humans we are 'hard wired' to observe others' states so we can more appropriately interact and empathise or manage the boundaries and this enables us to resonate with others, often at an unconscious level. When we experience leaders as 'authentic', we trust them more and when we trust our leaders our focus becomes more on improving the task at hand, which in turn improves performance. In addition, by sharing doubts and vulnerabilities in a way that allows connection with staff, staff are more willing and comfortable to offer advice and support, which in situations where we know that the higher up you go in an organisation the less likely you are to get honest feedback, which in turn means a more effective, productive and, in health settings, safer organisation (Larcker, 2013).

Example from Practice 3.7

Fiona, General Manager

Fiona was the General Manager for Women and Children's Services in a small district general hospital that was finding it increasingly difficult to meet the paediatric nurse-to-child ratio. There were a number of issues contributing to this including no facility for day casework and the current organising of paediatric surgery. The ward manager had repeatedly tried to attract staff to the unit with no luck and the pressure of the budgets was such that more strategic discussions had started about closing the inpatient unit. Fiona sat down with the staff and laid out all the issues as she saw them. She was totally honest about the potential risks but also stated that she thought reorganising how services were run could address the issues. The staff started to come up with a number of solutions, which included reorganisation of surgical lists. Fiona spoke to the general manager in surgery who said the surgeons were not happy to have anyone tell them how to run their lists and that they would not be prepared to change. Fiona gathered the data on a breakdown of surgical activity and the staffing issues and met with the lead surgeon, explaining that if they didn't change they would be facing closure of the paediatric unit. She asked the surgeon if he could help. The surgeon agreed to work with Fiona on a draft timetable to block children's surgery so that they could shift the staffing and meet the guidelines, which would also address some of the difficulties he was having in theatre. By being open with the staff about the difficulties and her inability to solve the issues on her own, Fiona was able to build the trust of the staff and together they came up with a solution that worked.

Often when we hear stories of how people behave, we move to value judgements and claims of what we would have done in that situation. Our estimate of what we would do in those situations can be easier to make when we are not actually caught in the grip of the emotional state.

The role of identity

> Who you are speaks so loudly I can't hear what you are saying.
>
> Ralph Waldo Emerson

When considering what factors influence who speaks up or not and how it is received, it is interesting to explore how people identify themselves or are identified by others. The stereotypes of the 'angelic' nurse or the 'difficult' consultant create a sense of identity which influences how people behave towards each other.

Koerner (2014) looked at the intersection of identity dynamics and workplace courage and suggests that in accounts of workplace courage, courageous behaviour is viewed as an important form of identity work that helps individuals to minimise any incongruence between that self and social identities.

Example from Scholarship 3.1

Workforce Modelling, Leary et al., 2016

Professor Alison Leary is a Professor of Workforce Modelling and has undertaken extensive research looking at the impact of the ratio of registered nurses to patients across a range of clinical areas (Leary et al., 2016). Her research supports the work of others (Griffiths et al., 2016 and Aitkin et al., 2017) which show that there is a relationship between the number of registered nurses and morbidity and mortality data (Leary et al., 2016). As a scientist by training, Alison describes how she is drawing on the data to show a relationship that many staff are sharing anecdotally from their lived experiences working in the clinical setting. With increasing shortages in nursing (estimated vacancies of 34,260 – NHS Digital, 2018), people are looking at ways of redesigning roles in the workforce to meet the changing demands of healthcare. This includes the use of technology and the introduction of new roles such as the physician's assistant and the nursing associate. Whilst acknowledging the need to look at ways of increasing staff, the balance of managing risk in vacancies needs to be balanced with the risk of having less experienced and educated staff looking after more complex and sicker patients. The introduction of nursing associates has raised concerns amongst the nursing profession and sits in the context of public perception around degree-educated nurses being less compassionate (Willis Commission, 2012). Yet the research on having degrees making you less compassionate isn't supported whilst the relationship between registered nurses and safety is. By speaking out publicly on this Alison and colleagues are openly challenging a direction of national policy, which in a highly 'political' context is not easy. But her identity as a scientist, as well as her professional responsibility as a nurse, and the evidence from the research, enable her to withstand criticism and any 'political' pressure.

Identity work in healthcare helps us to explore everyday acts of courage that are a normal part of organisational life and highlights the need to recognise the complexity and limitations of discerning identity(ies) and the interplay between organisational dynamics (Lopez et al., 2003).

It is important to recognise that people have multiple identities; this is particularly important in healthcare/social care where clinical/professionals take on extended managerial roles or others and how that begins to shape how they respond and are responded to when taking up a leadership stance (Dickenson et al., 2013; Limb, 2014).

This is not just in areas of taking up management but stepping outside of what are seen as roles and responsibilities that meet the perception of what a professional should or should not do. The introduction of Schwartz Rounds® across the NHS is quite a counter-cultural intervention, requiring staff to share and discuss emotions at work. They are facilitated by someone trained in group dynamics and psychological theory, and a medical consultant. Medical facilitators often share how they are very conscious of how their medical colleagues will receive them working with 'emotions' and non-solution focused activity as opposed to the more usual domain of scientific facts. This requires them to not only be courageous in stepping outside of the 'traditional' view of consultants but also in their role advocating this as important work, which traditionally has not been recognised but dismissed as 'touchy, feely'.

In looking at the role of identity theory in courage, how an individual defines themselves and their role plays a part in the undertaking of courageous acts. *Personal identity* describes a person's distinctive characteristics and self-definition, whereas *social identity* refers to who a person is in relation to a social entity (Pratt, 1998). We may have multiple identities in life generally as well as in organisations and this can result in us being pulled in different directions and having internal struggles about how to behave.

'Identity work' refers to the activities we engage in actively and continuously to create, preserve, repair and revise our identity in social contexts, the overall goal being to create a coherent and unique identity and manage the boundaries between personal and social (Alvesson and Willmott, 2002). 'Self' identity would be seen to be consistent across roles and situations but 'role' identity is tied to a person's position (Burke and Stets, 2009). Social identity is based on a person's membership in a salient group (e.g. a particular team, or organisation). This enables us to see people's behaviour and demonstration of courage in the context of their relational identity with others (Sluss and Ashforth, 2007). In this way, the courage to be who you are, even in a social context that wants or expects you to be different, requires emotional work and courage.

Workplace courage – why is it necessary?

Understanding organisations as 'complex social systems' helps us to appreciate the conditions that are created that influence how those within them and around them behave. These features of the workplace can coalesce to make courageous behaviour both necessary for organisational effectiveness and risky for individuals. Due to the nature of the work we require people with different backgrounds and perspectives to cooperate, which inevitably leads to power struggle and conflict (Clegg, 1989); whether that is advocating for minority positions, as well as speaking up about major organisational risks or corruption. The work of NHS England in implementing the NHS Workforce Race Equality Standard (WRES) (https://www.england.nhs.uk/about/equality/equality-hub/equality-standard/) led by people such as Yvonne Coghill, CBE, and Roger Kline looking at the experiences of staff from a BAME background in the NHS highlights this in the publication, *The 'snowy white peaks'* of the NHS (see: www.england.nhs.uk/wp-content/uploads/2014/08/edc7-0514.pdf).

In order for progress we need the development of innovative and entrepreneurial endeavours that enable organisations to thrive or take significant financial risk. This means disrupting the status quo and shifting existing power bases, patterns of behaviour and ways of relating. Work in itself is often a central feature of people's lives; it provides socio-economic, psychological and instrumental resources to people. Taking any form of courageous act that could threaten this can be far reaching at the personal, group, organisation and 'system' level. We explore this more in Chapter 5.

In healthcare, we would add a fourth which is the nature of the work itself and the emotional labour and courage to make oneself emotionally available to the physical and psychological distress of others, knowing that to do so makes one vulnerable, as referred to in Chapter 2.

All of these create a distinctive context for exploring courageous acts that occur in healthcare environments.

Described as one of the vital parts of work in organisational life, courage is often on the list of characteristics required by those in leadership roles and in leading (Lombardo and Eichinger, 2003; Kouzes and Posner, 2008). Acts of courage in this context are seen as oppositional behaviours such as constructive opposition to the status quo, for example 'positive deviance' (Sternin and Choo, 2000). Organisations are 'systems' that have established routines and control mechanisms often designed to maintain the status quo. Actions that challenge this are often met with resistance, even when they will improve organisational functioning. Courage is required to interrupt these patterns and the individual agency that goes with it – to be the one that questions, rather than simply accept. The design of organisations – be they hierarchical or bureaucratic (e.g. Laloux, 2014) – will influence the acts that require courage as some things will be promoted and others inhibited. These are sometimes implicit (unspoken norms and culture) or explicit (organisational policies or behavioural frameworks) and enabling people to undertake 'positively deviant' acts in the service of delivering good care is important.

When is courage *not* courage?

We would argue that acts that are done through coercion or chance are neither courageous nor bold and are more rash decisions that did not require deliberation (Cavanagh and Moberg, 1999).

Sometimes courage is demonstrated by not acting, such as resisting carrying out instructions that are seen as dangerous, unethical or unsafe, or biding time before saying anything despite high levels of personal distress.

The act is only considered courageous if it involves emotional difficulty, personal risks, threats and obstacles. The risks need to be significant (as defined by the person), such as loss of job, or friends, physical injury or, at the existential level, the courage to redefine oneself (Rollo, 1975). This could also include undertaking new roles or skills – which require new ways of being, thinking and being seen – as well as risky or challenging opportunities.

Example from Practice 3.8

Imperial Healthcare Trust

In the midst of concerns about the performance of the NHS, Imperial Healthcare NHS Trust allowed a Channel 4 film crew to deliver a documentary about life in a busy London teaching hospital. The programme showed the challenges of staff shortages, bed shortages and the daily difficulties staff and patients and their families faced. The programme had an average viewing figure of over 2.5 million and the public saw a realistic portrayal of issues around funding of the NHS, which did not present the government in a good light. This required courage of the Trust Board, staff and patients and their families to allow cameras to show everyone's vulnerability as well as their resolve in the face of adversity.

This exposure to the reality of delivering healthcare has challenged numerous perceptions around: safety; inefficiencies and attitudes of NHS staff. The public could now see the consequences of: staff shortages; insufficient beds and underfunding, exposing the impact of government decisions about the NHS. In a political system those who agreed to allow the filming might well have been anxious about repercussions and thus took a brave and courageous decision to agree to this.

Working away from the limelight

As we said at the beginning of this chapter, when considering those who are seen as 'courageous leaders', it is often those charismatic figures, publicly standing up for injustice and upholding ethical behaviour, making history and significant change that are cited. Yet, it is often those 'quiet leaders' who move patiently, carefully and incrementally righting, or preventing, moral wrongs in the workplace, inconspicuously and usually without casualties that make the biggest difference (Badaracco, 2001).

What is interesting to note is who gets quoted or seen as leading in this field and the style of different 'leaders' in getting their message across.

Quiet moral leaders tend to follow four basic rules:

1. *Putting things off till tomorrow* – Allows emotions to settle and stand back to see the interplay between different elements and patterns of behaviour before acting, to reduce the risk of problems further down the line.

2. *Picking their battles* – Not always charging in with a moral stand but being able to express a position that makes people rethink their own views or behaviours in a way that enables them to adjust rather than taking things head on.
3. *Bending the rules, not breaking them* – Looking at how to interpret rules in order to maximise the benefit to the core purpose.
4. *Finding a compromise* – Whilst this can often be seen as avoiding issues or 'doing a deal' quiet leaders realise that whilst moral approaches are important, taking the moral high ground is not. The work they do is crafting responsible, workable compromises that address the moral and ethical dilemmas faced.

Quiet moral leaders tend to typically work in the middle of organisations and are everyday folk trying to manage the often difficult 'middle' space of organisational life without seeking public recognition or glory. They often are not counselling perfection, and their thinking is distinguished by two characteristics: 'motivations which are decidedly mixed, and world views which are unabashedly realistic' (Badaracco, 2001). These 'mixed motivations' can create uncertainty and anxiety about what to do which, in itself, can lead people to pause and reflect before they act. It is often in the pausing and reflecting that people are able to make wise decisions. With regards to realistic views it is important to pay attention to the limits of your power and influence. Full-out whistleblowing (as we see in Chapter 5) can be career suicide and taking dramatic actions, which back others into a corner – especially if they have more power – rarely leads to a good outcome. Finding ways to work with the reality and options around can often be more effective in dealing with difficult organisational issues.

This often unnoticed and unglamorous activity of the quiet leader represents what keeps organisations on track every day, suggesting that it is not simply the dramatic efforts of people at the top, but the consistent striving of those working far from the limelight. When we look at the recent pressures in the NHS around A&E performance over winter, we see it is the everyday decisions of staff across health and social care that is allowing the organisations to continue to function and patients to receive the best care they can. Local negotiations by leaders to cut corners on paperwork, and policies and procedures to speed up decision making and share resources which benefit the people under these teams' care, require the courage to ignore national policy when required.

A role for moral philosophy?

Richard Kilberg (2012) explores the role of moral philosophy and how it is examined in leadership to be able to make a stand or make decisions guided by a moral compass. With the increased volatility of today's society, the need for people of virtue to direct organisations if they are to survive and thrive into the twenty-first century has never been greater. With the constant moral and ethical dilemmas that face those in health and social care in their everyday work, and the increased pressure of rising demand against diminishing resources, we would argue that significantly more attention and effort are required in this area if we are to navigate these times successfully. Thus having a 'moral compass' – which combines having a moral vision, a moral code, moral fitness and moral performance as a leader – is essential. This raises the issue of power, politics, influence, persuasion and leadership and the acquisition and use of power and influence and how these should be applied.

Aristotle argues the view that a leader (*aka* King) should listen and take advice of true philosophers, which, by doing so, would 'enrich his/her leadership (reign) with not only good words but more importantly good deeds (p17, 2009)'.

Values

It is useful to explore how leaders draw upon their values and articulate them as a blueprint for organisational behaviour. Frost (2014) explores a number of case studies to examine how 'values-based' leadership affects organisational performance. He looked at how different organisations develop and maintain a value-based culture. Values-based leadership requires leaders to be courageous as well as humble, as defining values, and all that comes from it, can lead to challenges of well entrenched behaviours which can lead to conflict. In addition, the examining and articulation of the leader's values, means that the values and leader are open to the scrutiny of consistent application and challenge if not followed. Alongside courage and humility, the main factors for enabling value-based leadership are whether leaders are willing to learn, whether they want to lead and whether they are able to deal with the change and ambiguity that exist in organisational life and an ever-changing environment (Frost, 2014). These constitute three dimensions of values-based leadership, outlined in Figure 3.3.

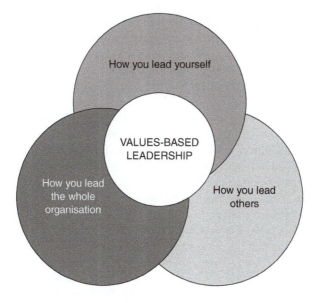

Figure 3.3   Values-based leadership model

Source: Adapted from Frost (2014)

It requires you to model constantly these values in everything you do. When these are in balance you get a sustainable and dynamic organisational culture that has the ability to change and create long-term repeatable success, emotional connection and the engagement of employees and customers of the organisation, the ability of the whole organisation to be responsive and adapt to the changing environment within which it operates, and leadership that wins the trust, respect and confidence of people in the organisation (Frost, 2014).

We think it is helpful to look at these three dimensions in more detail.

Leading self

This is not just what you believe, but how you behave – constantly. It requires you to constantly model those values in everything you do.

Knowing yourself and your values and moral compass to respond in a considered and balanced way – this is not always easy when under considerable pressure to respond.

Example from Practice 3.9

Jane, Senior Manager, District General Hospital

Jane was a senior manager in a District General Hospital (DGH) and the senior manager on call. Beds were tight and pressure on the emergency department (ED) meant the bed management team were pushing hard for discharges. One of the nursing team managing the complex discharges was very distressed about an elderly woman who was homeless that she had tried to organise accommodation for but with no luck, and had now been told needed to be discharged by the Chief Operating Officer (COO) even if she was homeless.

Jane was clear about her own values as well as what the Chief Executive (CEO) described as hers. She was also aware of the pressure the COO was under and of his behaviour, which, at times, made others anxious and reluctant to challenge him. Jane knew that if this situation was not challenged the nurse would not believe it was a value-driven organisation and also would not feel able to challenge in future if asked to do the same thing. Jane knew the strength of her on-going relationship lay in an alignment of the nurse's values on doing the right thing for this patient with Jane's own and that her behaviour was the indication of this. Jane also knew she had to model what she wanted the nurse to do in future. Jane spoke to the COO and said it was clearly not good care to discharge this patient onto the street and that she would work with the local council and voluntary sector to find a temporary home until a permanent arrangement was found. She told him that his involvement would indicate the importance of this issue with housing colleagues to find a positive outcome for the patient and all organisations. The COO agreed and made several calls, which resulted in a charity providing shelter. He then found Jane and the nurse to tell them he had resolved it, which enabled him to be seen in a more favourable light and the nurse to feel that her role as advocate of patients was one that was valued.

Leading others

Leading others means helping groups to agree how to work together with each other and develop a mutual sense of respect and support, through collaboration and understanding of their interdependency.

Example from Practice 3.10

Cynthia, Medical Director

Cynthia was the newly appointed medical director of an acute hospital who was looking to strengthen the participation and challenge of the consultant body. Clinical director roles had been taken up either as a way to argue the case for individual departments or 'because no one else wanted to do it'. Cynthia knew that what would make the organisation successful was clinical leaders who would critically analyse decisions and be willing to take and defend difficult decisions which were in the interest of patients and the whole organisation, not just one department, and she needed to build a team amongst the existing group. Several of the group had not wanted Cynthia to be the medical director and had been openly critical of her in the past. This required a building and repairing of relationships which had broken down due to mistrust and operational pressures.

Over a one-year programme, Cynthia worked with her team and an outside facilitator to share who they were as individuals and what their core values were. They learnt how to share frustrations and disputes and deal with issues that had been bubbling for years. They learnt how to disagree with each other, including how to challenge Cynthia, and to work through differences to reach positions that all felt able to work with and to become a strong and effective team. Whilst uncomfortable for Cynthia, as not only a woman in a male-dominated group but also someone from a Black, Minority, Ethnic group (BME) who had experienced both sexism and racism in the organisation, she was determined that the values of excellence in care and respectful debate and dialogue were at the core of the team's functioning which meant challenging each other was fundamental. Using various frameworks such as the Thomas Kilmann Inventory and other psychometric tools, the team gained deep insight into their own and each other's

(Continued)

(Continued)

beliefs and behaviours, which enabled them to accept their own and others' strengths and weaknesses and draw on them when required. This emphasised the independency between them and enabled them to compensate for individual weaknesses in team members.

This leadership group became a powerful voice and, as they gained confidence in their own competence and effectiveness, they were more able to challenge the executive team about operational decisions and lead internal operations so that the executive team could focus on their critical role of strategy and external relationships, enhancing the overall effectiveness of all the senior leadership teams.

Leading the organisation

At an organisational level, this is making sure the values align with the purpose of the organisation. Far too often, organisations have values, which are placed on posters across the organisation, which bear little resemblance to the culture and behaviours in the organisation or align with the strategy of the organisation. This misalignment creates conflict and tension as people experience incongruence between what is espoused and what is enacted (Schein, 2010). When this is the case, reference to values can actually do more harm than good.

Courage to be 'different'

Courage is not always about speaking up, but sometimes about being different.

Example from Practice 3.11

Rob, CEO of Bromley by Bow Centre

Rob Trimble is the CEO of the Bromley by Bow Centre (see www.bbbc.org.uk) which has been increasingly cited as a model for organising what people in the NHS refer to as local 'place-based' healthcare. Visited by significant numbers of health leaders and international health communities, the work they have done on supporting the local community to address the wider determinates of health, rather than the medical model, has been described as a blue-print for the future and something to be replicated across the UK. Rob and his team have an interesting business model, which has both charitable status and statutory healthcare funding, and provides financial and business support to a large number of start-up businesses run by local entrepreneurs. But Rob and the team are conscious of the uniqueness of the centre in terms of how it came about and the history which enabled it to evolve into what it is today.

The request by policy makers and senior leaders across the NHS to expand and replicate the model, as well as act as an advisor to others, is flattering and seductive and yet also a challenge to what Rob believes should happen through community-led development, which is organic in nature and evolves as communities build effective relationships and organise themselves to create services that support them.

In addition, in expanding, there is also a challenge to the 'appropriate' size and scale of the Bromley by Bow Centre, which has been successful due to its local focus and strong community involvement and connections.

Working in an environment where 'scale and pace' are heavily promoted, Rob knows that these relationships take time and are strengthened by the relatively small size where people can have meaningful relationships.

In an environment where models of care are defined centrally and then advocated across all settings, the ability to go against the grain and form your own path can be met with criticism.

Following the Transforming Community Services (2008), Community Trusts were offered the opportunity to join with existing hospital-based services or establish independent organisations.

Example from Practice 3.12

Siobhan Clarke, nurse professional

Siobhan Clarke is a nurse professional and the Managing Director of Your HealthCare. Siobhan led the externalisation of Provider Services from Kingston Primary Care Trust (PCT) working with staff to develop a successful bid to become a mutual co-operative social enterprise in 2010, forming a Community Interest Company which is a not for profit organisation where any surplus is re-invested into services and the local community. Siobhan was one of the very few who managed to secure an NHS pension for her staff as they transferred into the social enterprise and has continued to push at the edge of policy to develop new ways of working. They have had integrated health and social care teams since it began in 2010 without any national transformation funded teams. Staff at the organisation have local discretionary budgets, which enable them to make spot purchases for things that will make a difference to patients' lives, from equipment to microwaves, to promote independence.

This deep understanding of local 'systems' of care and the communities they serve means these leaders can work at the right size and speed of the quality of the relationships. Failure to understand your local context, and a single minded focus on achieving rapid and effective change to ensure improvements in organisational performance, is often met with a lack of response from 'front line' staff and becomes a barrier to effective change.

Courage to be human

Real change and transformation takes place when leaders manage the human dimensions of the change process with great care – often dismissed as the 'soft stuff'. Whilst this has been recognised and written about for many decades, we still see job specifications for those in leadership roles with management, business or finance as essential criteria, rather than human and organisational psychology.

The role of courage in patient safety

When considering the importance of addressing safety concerns in healthcare and what prevents people from speaking up, and applying the approaches developed, the main barrier is interpersonal which is influenced by the moral courage of individuals to take action in the face of concerns (Geller, 2009). Whilst competence and commitment to act are important, without moral courage competence and commitment alone will not be sufficient.

Example from Practice 3.13

Hannah, community nurse

Hannah was a community nurse working on a late shift. She and a colleague had been called to see a patient who was dying and was in pain. When they arrived Hannah realised that the medication for the syringe driver had been written incorrectly and they could not set it up. They needed the out-of-hours GP to visit and review the patient. Whilst Hannah gave a stat dose of analgesia, her colleague called the GP but was diverted to 111 to speak to a call handler. They explained they were the District Nursing Team and the situation and asked to be put straight through to the GP but were told they had to answer a number of questions first. On answering it became clear that she couldn't answer them and

---

the call handler asked to speak to the patient. The nurse reiterated the situation with the patient and the handler then insisted they spoke to the relative. The colleague handed over the phone to the relative who answered the first few questions and then became increasingly distressed. With the patient now settled, Hannah took the phone and asked to speak to the GP. Initially the call handler refused. Due to Hannah's experience and knowledge of what was needed she said she would not answer any more questions and that the call handler was to either put her through or she would be making a formal complaint that they were delaying treatment to a terminally ill patient. The call was put through and the GP initially was abrupt and irritated that the prescription was inadequate. They asked Hannah to just administer the 'correct' dosage. Hannah refused saying this wasn't correct practice, she had only just met the patient and had very little background information as she did not have access to the GP notes. She also knew that the GP had a duty of care and was obliged to visit and thus stayed firm in her insistence that the GP visit and assess the patient.

With the patient settled they left with a commitment that the GP would visit within the next hour, and advised the family to contact the district nurses if there were any further problems.

In Example from practice 3.12, was not just the courage to stand up to the 'system' but also Hannah's knowledge of what was required and the GP's professional responsibility that enabled her to insist on action. Whilst courage is a human characteristic distinct from commitment and competence, these three qualities of leadership are interdependent (Geller, 2009). Specifically, individuals with greater competence and commitment in a given situation are more likely to demonstrate courage. One's propensity to show courage under certain circumstances is increased whenever the relevant competence or commitment is augmented.

Example from Practice 3.14

Steven, NHS Consultant

Steven was an experienced consultant with over 30 years in the NHS. A strong advocate for the importance of education and training, he had been appointed to be the lead for medical education in a large internationally renowned teaching hospital.

(Continued)

(Continued)

His story gives a sense of the difficulties that he encountered and the feelings of being torn by a strong sense of duty and loyalty.

Already facing significant revenue challenges, the organisation was struggling to meet the requirements for achieving Foundation Trust Status (in 2003) and was drawing heavily on private patient, overseas and charitable funds to balance their budget.

A recent clinical case had been attracting significant media and political interest, and the long standing CEO was experiencing a diminution of internal support from clinical teams due to a series of difficult and therefore unpopular decisions.

At the same time, there was a national re-organisation occurring in education with the introduction of a policy to modernise medical careers (2005) that was having a backlash from the medical profession around the impact on the quality of training and service provision.

As the lead for medical education with responsibility for implementing the recommended changes to medical workforce and training, Steven was trying to balance a number of competing demands. Over this time he became increasingly concerned about plans for a reduction in junior doctors and the knock-on effect on rotas.

As someone with an eye for detail and evidence-based practice, Steven recognised the importance of meticulously capturing data to assess the impact of changes and the need to carry out comprehensive risk assessments to inform decision making. He was fastidious in keeping an audit trail of communication with relevant stakeholders to ensure risks were identified, escalated where necessary, and in mitigating plans discussed, agreed and monitored to enable plans to be adjusted accordingly.

Steven became increasingly concerned about the level of post reductions being proposed to reduce workforce costs, and flagged this with the CEO and relevant workforce committee, submitting a report offering alternative approaches, which would deliver some of the cost reduction whilst maintaining a 'safe' rota. This was not received favourably and the response was to recruit a senior project manager to lead the change. Steven felt sidelined and undermined. This was the first experience of many that was to test his resilience.

As his level of concern increased he submitted an email to the CEO, copied to the executive team, which included data on an increased level of critical incidents being reported due to gaps in junior doctor rotas, and offered recommendations for improvement.

Simultaneously there was a backlash from medical colleagues regarding the impact of junior doctor training on service provision, leading to discussions of a vote of no

confidence in the CEO. Pressure was also mounting from regulators to meet FT requirements and a serious incident was being investigated by the media, the Department of
Health and the Secretary of State for Health.

Steven tried to defend the CEO to the consultant body, outlining the pressures
within the wider 'system', and appealed to them to look for solutions to the problems of a tightening financial landscape and changes in medical training and workforce gaps. Despite this, it became increasingly clear, from interactions with fellow
executives, that his continued raising of concerns and alternative proposals was
causing difficulties. Steven was spoken to by the medical director and asked to
relinquish his role in education to focus on service commitment in an area that was
known to be underfunded and struggling. For Steven this was another act of
undermining and withdrawal of his ability to influence. He began to notice the
effects on his mental health and wellbeing and the need for support from friends
and trusted colleagues.

Recognising his position was feeling increasingly untenable he was approached
by colleagues in a different organisation to lead a new service. A compromise
agreement was offered which Steven's lawyers advised him on and whilst he found
it difficult to initially accept, he realised that he was unable to effect the change
required or stay without speaking up about his concerns. Ironically as the agreement was signed, the original concerns were validated by the external project
team and subsequent medical lead. For Steven, whilst personally adversely
affected, he felt able to leave knowing the risks to patient care and junior doctors'
wellbeing were being mitigated, and so the compromise agreement was signed
and Steven left.

Following his departure, Steven became unwell and was prescribed a course of anti-
depressants but, with the support of friends, family and colleagues, was able to rebuild
a successful and impactful career.

Several years later, the same organisation was facing renewed public interest in a
difficult case with criticism of the CEO in the handling of concerns of safety that had
been raised. Steven was approached by health officials and new executives at the
organisation about concerns he had raised previously which were part of public
documents. He knew his comments could be extremely damaging to the organisation and the CEO but could also cause difficulties for his new organisation and his
specialty.

With numerous requests from journalists, Steven was being given an opportunity
to not only be publicly vindicated from previous slurs about him but also to 'right' an
injustice. After much soul searching and assurances from relevant parties that the
situation would be effectively managed, he decided not to speak to the media and in
doing so describes how he was able to let go of the anger and distress the experience
had caused.

Our propensity to take a courageous act can be understood by drawing on the five person states model which looks at the psychological states needed to be present for someone to 'actively' care, i.e. act upon their concerns (Geller, 2009) (see Figure 3.4). When these states are attended to and the cultural factors of organisational life that develop and cultivate daily acts of courage by co-workers are in place (see Chapter 6), people will act.

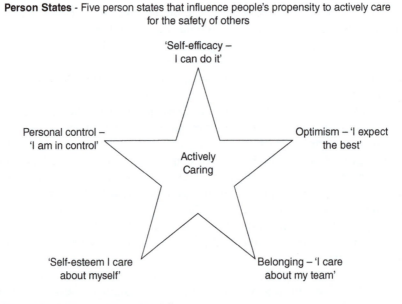

Person States - Five person states that influence people's propensity to actively care for the safety of others

'Self-efficacy – I can do it'

Personal control – 'I am in control'

Optimism – 'I expect the best'

Actively Caring

'Self-esteem I care about myself'

Belonging – 'I care about my team'

Figure 3.4   Geller's 'Person States Model'

Source: Adapted from the work of Geller (e.g. 1996)

Creating opportunities for people to voluntarily join conversations about safety and errors in an environment that is designed for learning can enhance the opportunity for others to follow. Whilst most safety leaders are competent and committed regarding the application of cost-effective interventions to prevent injuries, without the moral courage to step up and take an interpersonal risk, action will not occur. Using the 'person states' model to understand the contributory factors that influence individual acts of courage (self-esteem, belongingness, personal control, self-efficacy and optimism) could be very helpful to the individual intervening in the system in a morally courageous way. Therefore, leaders need to create environments that increase these person states amongst themselves, and others, to enhance the courage to intervene when required. We return to this in Chapter 6.

Lessons for us all?

This chapter starts to guide the reader into seeing things from different angles in the hope that acts that are deemed as courageous, or not, are given a wider understanding with the purpose of encouraging others to act when required. It is important to see this not just as an act of bravery or courage – which raises the intensity of the situation and level of fear – but more as something that is an everyday occurrence and is important for the greater good of the NHS and the people we serve. Starting to see this behaviour in everyday colleagues as well as those in formal positions of leadership provides confidence and competence in us all to take action and to truly behave in what Michael West and colleagues (2014) describe as 'collective leadership'.

Useful Weblinks

www.good-governance.org.uk/wp-content/uploads/2017/04/Good-Governance-Hand book.pdf
https://chfg.org/trustees/martin-bromiley
www.leadingtoday.org/changing-toxic-organizational-culture
www.ted.com/talks/brene_brown_on_vulnerability
See NIHR Evaluation of Schwartz Rounds at: www.nihr.ac.uk/blogs/how-can-we-support-healthcare-staff-to-care-well-a-national-evaluation-of-schwartz-center-rounds/7765

References

Aitkin, L.H., Sloane, D., Griffiths, P., Rafferty, A.M., Bruyneel, L., McHugh, M., Maier, C.B., Moreno-Casbas, T., Ball, J.E., Ausserhofer, D. and Sermeus, W. (2017) 'Nursing skill mix in European hospitals: Cross-sectional study of the association with mortality, patient ratings, and quality of care', *BMJ Quality & Safety*, 26(7): 559–568.

Alimo-Metcalfe, B., Bradley, M., Alban-Metcalfe, J. and Locker, A. (2013) 'Leading to quality: An investigation of the impact of leadership & team working on staff morale and wellbeing, and team performance, among mental health teams within Yorkshire and the Humber Strategic Health Authority', University of Bradford School of Management.

Alvesson, M. and Willmott, H. (2002) 'Identity regulation as organizational control: Producing the appropriate individual', *Journal of Management Studies*, 39(5): 619–644.

Andrews, M. (2013) *Going Beyond Heroic-leaders in Development*. Cambridge, MA: Center for International Development at Harvard University.

Aristotle, with Ross,W.D. and Brown, L. (2009) *The Nicomachean Ethics*. Oxford: Oxford University Press.

Badaracco, J. (2001) 'We don't need another Hero', *Harvard Business Review*, 79(8): 120–126.

Bailey, J. (2012) *From Ward to Whitehall: the Disaster at Mid Staffs*. Stafford: Cure the NHS.

Bailey, J. (2014) 'Cure the NHS', *Clinical Psychology Forum 263*. Available at: www1.bps.
org.uk/system/files/user-files/Division%20of%20Clinical%20Psychology/public/cpf263_
extended_final.pdf (accessed 1 June 2018).

Berne, E. (1964) *Games People Play: The Psychology of Human Relationships*. London:
Penguin.

Brown, B. (2015) *Daring Greatly: How the Courage to Be Vulnerable Transforms the Way
We Live, Love, Parent and Lead*. New York: Avery Publishing Group.

Buber, M. (1923) *I and Thou*. London: Continuum.

Burke, P.J. and Stets, J.E. (2009) *Identity Theory*. Oxford: Oxford University Press.

Cavanagh, G.F. and Moberg, D.J. (1999) 'The virtue of courage within the organization',
Research in Ethical Issues in Organizations, 1: 1–25.

Chaleff, I. (2009) *The Courageous Follower: Standing up to and for our Leaders*. San
Francisco, CA: Berrett-Koehler Publishers.

Challeff, I. (2015) *Intelligenct Disobedience: Doing Right When You're Told to Do Wrong*.
Oakland, CA: Berrett-Koehler.

Chambers, N., Harvey, G., Mannion, R., Bond, J. and Marshall, J. (2013) 'Towards a framework for enhancing the performance of NHS Boards: a synthesis of the evidence about
board governance, board effectiveness and board development', *Health Services and
Delivery Research*. doi:10.3310/hsdr01060.

Clegg, S.R. (1989) 'Radical revisions: Power, discipline and organizations', *Organization
Studies*, 10(1): 97–115.

Cook, A.F. and Hoas, H. (2008) 'Ethics and rural healthcare: What really happens? What
might help?', *American Journal of Bioethics*, 8(4): 52–56.

Dickenson, H., Ham, C. and Snelling, P. (2013) *Are We There Yet? Models of Medical
Leadership and Their Effectiveness: An Exploratory Study*. National Institute of Health
Research Service Delivery and Organisational Programme.

Ellis, L. (2014) Identifying the four D's of dysfunctional leadership. Available at: www.sbnonline.
com/article/lee-ellis-identifying-the-four-d-s-of-dysfunctional-leaders (accessed, July 2018).

Finfgeld, D.L. (1999) 'Courage as a process of pushing beyond the struggle', *Quality Health
Researcrh'* 9(6): 803–814.

Frost, J. (2014) 'Values based leadership', *Industrial and Commercial Training*, 46(3):
124–129.

Garratt, B. (2010) *The Fish Rots from the Head: The Crisis in our Boardrooms – Developing
the Crucial Skills of the Competent Director*. London: Profile Books.

Geller, S.E. (2009) 'Courage, culture and interpersonal intervention: Practical, evidence-based
strategies for injury prevention', *Professional Safety*, 54(5): 43–51.

Goldberg, C. and Simon, J. (1982) 'Toward a psychology of courage: Implications for the
change (healing) process', *Journal of Contemporary Psychotherapy*, 13(2): 107–128.

Griffiths, P., Ball, J., Drennan, J., Dall'Ora, C., Jones, J., Maruotti, A., Popem, C., Recio
Saucedo, A. and Simon, M. (2016) 'Nurse staffing and patient outcomes: Strengths and
limitations of the evidence to inform policy and practice: A review and discussion paper
based on evidence reviewed for the National Institute for Health and Care Excellence Safe
Staffing Guideline Development', *International Journal of Nursing Studies*, 63: 213–225.

Harbour, M. and Kisfalvi, V. (2014) 'In the eye of the beholder: An exploration of managerial
courage', *Journal of Business Ethics*, 119: 493–515.

Hefferman, M. (2011) *Wilful Blindness: Why we Ignore the Obvious at our Peril*. New York:
Walker & Co.

Heider, F. (1958) *The Psychology of Interpersonal Relations*. New York: Wiley.

Iles, V. (2005) *Managing Change in the NHS*, 2nd edn Maidenhead: Open University Press.

Janis, I.L. (1982) *Groupthink: Psychological Studies of Policy Decisions and Fiascoes*. Boston: Houghton Mifflin.

Kilberg, R. (2012) *Virtuous Leaders: Strategy, Character and Influence in the 21st Century*. Washington, DC: American Psychological Association.

Kilmann, R.H., O'Hara, L.A. and Strauss, J.P. (2011) *Organizational Courage Assessment*. Newport Coast, CA: Kilmann Diagnostics.

Kline, R. (2014) *The Snowy White Peaks of the NHS: A Survey of Discrimination in Governance and Leadership and the Potential Impact on Patient Care in London and England*. Middlesex Business School. Available at: www.england.nhs.uk/wp-content/uploads/2014/08/edc7-0514.pdf (accessed 1 June 2018).

Koerner, M.M. (2014) 'Courage as identity work: Accounts of workplace courage', *Academy of Management Journal*, 57(1): 63–93.

Kouzes, J.M. and Posner, B.Z. (2008) *The Leadership Challenge: How to Make the Extraordinary Things Happen in Organisations* (4th edn). San Francisco, CA: Jossey Bass.

Larcker, D. (2013) *'Lonely at the Top' Resonates for Most CEOs*. Available at: www.gsb.stanford.edu/insights/david-larcker-lonely-top-resonates-most-ceos (accessed, July 2018).

Laloux, F. (2014) *Reinventing Organisations: A Guide to Creating Organizations Inspired by the Next Stage in Human Consciousness*. Brussels, Belgium: Nelson Parker.

Leary, A., Cook, R., Jones, S., Smith, J., Gough, M., Maxwell, E., Punshon, G. and Radford, M. (2016) 'Mining routinely collected data to reveal non-linear relationships between nurse staffing levels and outcomes', *BMJ*, 6(12).

Limb, M. (2014) 'What is deterring doctors from management roles', *BMJ Careers, 348*: g2785.

Lombardo, M. and Eichinger, R. (2003) *FYI: For Your Improvement – A Guide for Development and Coaching* (4th edn). Minnepolis, MN: Lominger Ltd, Inc.

Lopez, S.J., Koetting O'Byrne, K. and Peterson, S. (2003) 'Profiling courage in S.J. Lopez and C.R. Synder (eds), *Positive Psychological Assessment: A Handbook of Models and Measures*. Washington: American Psychological Association pp. 185–197.

NHS Digital (2018) https://digital.nhs.uk/data-and-information/publications/statistical/nhs-vacancies-survey/nhs-vacancy-statistics-england-february-2015-september-2017-provisional-experimental-statistics

Powell, A. and Davies, H. (2016) *Managing Doctors, Doctors Managing*. Nuffield Trust.

Pratt, M.G. (1998), To be or not to be: Central questions in organizational identification. in D.A. Whetten and P.C. Godfrey (eds), *Foundations for Organizational Science: Identity in Organizations Building Theory through Conversations*. Thousand Oaks, CA: Sage, pp. 171–207.

Rollo, M. (1975) *The Courage to Create*. New York: W.W. Norton.

Ross, L. (1977) 'The intuitive psychologist and his shortcomings: Distortions in the attribution process', in L. Berkowitz, *Advances in Experimental Social Psychology*. New York: Academic Press. pp. 173–220.

Schein, E. (2010) *Organisational Culture and Leadership*. New York: Wiley.

Searle, R., Legood, A. and Teoh, K. (2014) *Trust Boards and Governance: Composition and Behavioural Styles in Implementing Culture Change within the NHS – Contributions from Occupational Psychology*. London: British Psychological Society.

Senge, P. (1999) *The Dance of Change: The Challenges of Sustaining Momentum in Learning Organisations*. London: Nicholas Brealey Publishing.

Sluss and Ashforth (2007) 'Relational identity and identification: Defining ourselves through work relations', *Academy of Management Review*, 32(1): 9–32.

Sternin, J. and Choo, R. (2000) 'The power of positive deviancy', *Harvard Business Review*, 78(1).

Sutton, R. (2007) *The No Asshole Rule*. London: Sphere Publishing.

Transforming Community Services National Archives. Department of Health. *Archived from the original on* 3 May 2012. Retrieved March 2018.

Van Boven, L., Loewensteing, G., Welch, E. and Dunning, D. (2005) 'The illusion of courage in social predictions: Underestimating the impact of fear of embarrassment on other people', *Organisational Behaviour and Human Decision Processes*, 96: 130–141.

Walker, N. (n.d.) *Changing Toxic Organisational Culture*. Available at www.leadingtoday.org/changing-toxic-organizational-culture (accessed March 2018).

West, D. (2010) 'Lansley tells Confed: NHS needs strong Management', *Health Service Journal*, 24th February.

West, M.A., Lyubovnikova, R.E. and Denis, J.L. (2014) 'Collective leadership for cultures of high quality health care', *Journal of Organizational Effectiveness, People and Performance*, 1(3): 240–260.

Willis Commission (2012) *Quality with Compassion: The Future of Nursing Education*. Available at: www.williscommission.org.uk (accessed April 2018).

Worline, M.C. and Quinn, R. (2003) 'Courage at work: The interrelationship of organisational form and principled action', in K. Cameron, J. Dutton and R. Quinn (eds), *Positive Organizational Scholarship*. San Francisco, CA: Berrett-Koehler. pp. 138–157.

Younie, L. (2016) 'Vulnerable leadership', *London Journal of Primary Care*, 8(3): 37–38.

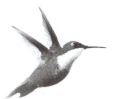

4

COURAGE TO LIVE AND DIE

SHIBLEY RAHMAN

Success is not final, failure is not fatal: it is the courage to continue that counts.

Winston Churchill

The phenomenon of courage in living and dying has been explored in philosophy, theology, literature, and other fields of inquiry mainly rooted in the humanities. An issue is to bridge this with the experiences within health and social care. Previous research has not often been directed toward a description and exploration of courage, although coping, compassion, caring and other experiences integral to the clinician–patient relationship have been examined. The holistic view of the complex effect of interacting influences on the individual patient is often overlooked. Life experiences during the course of life, anticipating death and reacting to someone's death are complex, and are not easily reducible in the phrase 'patient opinion'. Over the past centuries, efforts to construct a socially relevant view of courage have seen it go from the heart of the brave soldier on the battlefield to the experience of daily life and the mind of every person (Lopez et al., 2003). 'Never underestimate the importance of courage, confidence, and leadership ability to convene and hold challenging conversations in healthcare' (Meyer, 2014: 108).

Tillich (1952) recognised courage as an essential part of 'one's being'. And indeed courage appears to be, intuitively, an existential component for all of us.

Courage has been identified with resilience, particularly in recovery from intense suffering such as that experienced in the Holocaust (Tee, 2003). Courage has also been related to the search for 'meaning' in one's life (Frankl, 1939). Courage was linked to self-respect in remaining true to one's most enduring values by Kennedy (1955) in the now-classic *Profiles in Courage*.

The presence of fear has been noticeable in the analysis of life experiences. For example, Woodard (2004) identified courageous people as those who, despite perceiving a danger or threat beyond which their resources are capable of effectively managing, move forward and act anyway. This might be, for example, a reaction to being personally diagnosed with dementia or cancer. Gould (2005) likewise underlined that courage allows one to effectively act under conditions of danger, fear and risk. And yet it is appreciated that 'to live well' it is necessary to embrace some degree of risk. Finally, using a behavioural approach, Norton and Weiss (2009) stated that courage is distinct from fearlessness in that the courageous individual completes the same act as the fearless individual, despite experiencing fear.

The 'battle' analogy and the 'war against dementia'

The perception of living with a long-term condition has become strongly framed by the popular media as well as the specialist scientific press.

In particular, the history of the use and definition of metaphors can be traced back 2400 years when Aristotle described metaphor in his *Poetics* as 'giving the thing a name that belongs to something else' (McKeon, 1941: 1476). Metaphors have been described as a 'lens', providing us with special insights and data about the narrator and his or her emotions, beliefs and self-concepts, which are often unconsciously produced. Metaphors have been used about diseases and illnesses, and are fundamental to patients in perceiving, interpreting and defining symptoms, and motivating them to seek care (Johannessen et al., 2015).

When, for example, will we know when the 'war against dementia' is over? This is not an altogether frivolous question, as an MP once famously asked Tony Blair in Prime Minister's Questions: 'When will the war against terrorism be over?' On 28 November 2013, about dementia, Jeremy Hunt had written in *The Telegraph* about dementia: 'It is a truly horrible disease'. This set the 'mood music' for some of the G8 dementia conference. In *The Loss of Sadness*, Horwitz and Wakefield (2007) wrote that, while a depressive disorder can certainly be a devastating condition warranting medical attention, the apparent 'epidemic' in modern culture reflects the way the psychiatric profession (perhaps under the influence of pharmaceutical companies looking to widen markets) has understood and reclassified normal human sadness in the *DSM-IV* as a 'largely abnormal experience'.

The popular metaphorical framing of illness as a fight, war or battle seems to operate on various levels. Dementia is generalised as a vast, natural or monstrous force that we must 'fight', and it is also located as a very specific condition that affects individuals in extreme ways. In both cases, the effect can make us feel both terrified and relatively powerless. As the late Sir Terry Pratchett OBE said: 'People seem to think of Alzheimer's as something rather terrible and dreadful, almost as if witchcraft is involved' (Zeilig, 2014). Literally meaning 'away' or 'out' of 'mind' or 'reason' in Latin, the actual term 'dementia' entered the English language from the French *demence* via the French psychiatrist Philippe Pinel, who made notable contributions to the categorisation of mental disorders in the late eighteenth and early nineteenth centuries. Over the centuries, the phenomenology of dementia has been causally associated with witchcraft, moral degeneracy, bad blood and a dissipation of vital energy from the brain, among other factors.

David Cameron's opening to his speech at the G8 summit at Lancaster House on 11 December 2013 is interesting:

> It doesn't matter whether you're in London or Los Angeles, in rural India or urban Japan – this disease steals lives; it wrecks families; it breaks hearts and that is why all of us here are so utterly determined to beat it.

What kind of disease is it which steals, wrecks and breaks? This is the fundamental problem. Dementia is not a creature, it's not an alien, it's not a mega monster even and, whilst the use of this language can attract attention and thus funding for research, many functions remain in the early stages, which is why it can seem unfair to use such graphic language which leaves those affected potentially terrified and devoid of hope.

Medical and scientific discourses also tend to conflate dementia with crisis. Analysing some of the cultural scripts about dementia and Alzheimer's disease helps to reveal the underlying assumptions that infuse the political, social and medical narratives that are told about these conditions (Zeilig, 2014). Media have a central role in setting the agenda with regard to what is to be discussed and what is known at both the personal and political levels in relation to a variety of important social issues (e.g. Meissner et al., 1992).

Jeremy Hunt in *The Telegraph* had written:

> In the Sixties people were too scared to talk about cancer. In the Eighties, the same happened with HIV/Aids. After a long and painful journey, we are now much more open about both – and better able to tackle them.

It seems that this parallel with HIV/AIDS and cancer has been very carefully choreographed. There are indeed some successful treatments for many cancers, but cancer like dementia is an umbrella term covering a wide variety of conditions. A 'cure for dementia' is meaningless as a term, as the frontotemporal dementias particularly common in the younger age group are a different pathological entity to the most common type, the dementia of the Alzheimer type.

For most of us, the word dementia like Alzheimer's disease can invoke a profound dread. Dementia has replaced cancer as 'the scourge of modern times' (Van Gorp and Vercruysse, 2012: 1274). The discourses of the scientific community reinforce this pervasive sense of horror about dementia and Alzheimer's disease. For example, the prevalence of dementias is described in dramatic terms as an 'epidemic' and a 'crisis' (Mandell and Green, 2011: 4). The discourses of the scientific community reinforce this pervasive sense of horror about the dementias. For example, the prevalence of dementias is described in dramatic terms as an 'epidemic'. Flooding is a particular popular literary turn. The danger of flooding has long been associated with dementia. A 1982 UK report was entitled *The Rising Tide: Developing Services for Mental Illness in Old Age* (Health Advisory Service, 1982). Rising tides continue to inform the language of contemporary politicians when discussing dementia.

'Fight' is THE BIG prominent word. This recurring linguistic device in the cultural framing of dementia is the reliance on military and war-like metaphors. The dementia 'time bomb' crops up frequently in UK broadsheets and other tabloids. Time bombs are devices that could go off at any time; their most common use has been in politically motivated terrorism. The association of dementia with terrorist tactics is fascinating, invoking the sense of a threat.

The 'war against cancer'

Cancer has been described as the most feared of modern diseases (e.g. Beach et al., 2005). It has been associated with death, with long and sickening treatments, with punishment, a lack of cleanliness, contagion, unpredictability and traitorousness (Peters-Golden, 1982), among other things. Fear has led people with cancer to be stigmatised and isolated from social life (Fife and Wright, 2000). Stigmatisation results in diminished social status, negative self-perceptions and emotional well-being, social rejection, as well as limitations in employment opportunities (Link and Streuning, 1997). In 2010, Barbara Ehrenreich observed that breast cancer had become 'the biggest disease on the cultural map, bigger than AIDS, cystic fibrosis, or spinal injury, bigger even than those more prolific killers of women such as heart disease, lung cancer and stroke' (p. 45). In the dozen years since the publication of her controversial essay, the scrutiny of the actual lived experience of cancer has not diminished. This dominance makes itself felt in a variety of ways, such as in the visibility of breast cancer in the media (Seale, 2002).

Earlier investigations of the portrayal of cancer in the media have noted that the disease has been described as 'an evil and immoral predator', as an 'enemy' treated through military tactics, as leading to an 'untrustworthy' and 'suspect' body, as associated with death, fear and hopelessness, and as potentially caused by almost everything (Clarke, 1992). Military metaphors are widely used when describing health status and illness, and the mainstream media are frequently accused of perpetuating them. Military metaphors are certainly prevalent in newspaper headlines, in reference to a broad range of medical conditions including heart disease, obesity, multiple sclerosis, depression and allergies (Lane et al., 2013). When military metaphors predominate, the outcome of an illness becomes one of victory or defeat and hence both the diagnosis and prognosis are obligated to be binary phenomena. If someone does not 'win their battle' with illness, have they failed? The implication is that perhaps a person who is dying did not fight hard enough.

War on cancer was popularised in the 1970s through advertisements that initiated fear as a way of generating support for cancer research funding. A famous military reference to cancer was made by the US President Nixon in 1971 where cancer was referred to as a 'battle' or a 'war' to be fought and an illness to be killed. By waging war on cancer, resources were harnessed and protocols bypassed to ensure that the president was involved in cancer control efforts (Woodgate and Busolo, 2017). In a recent study, qualitative interviews with 14 informants (aged 18–30 years; nine daughters, five sons) were conducted in 2014, and subsequently analysed by the informants' use of metaphors. Steger's three-step method for analysing metaphors was applied. The analysis identified four themes in the metaphors: the informants' relations to the disease, to the self, to the parent, and to others. From these themes, four core metaphors were abstracted: 'my parent is sliding away'; 'emotional chaos'; 'becoming a parent to my parent'; and 'a battle' (Johannessen et al., 2015).

But what happens if you 'live through' a serious condition? If breast cancer has become the paradigm for understanding cancer 'survivorship' (life with and beyond cancer) more broadly, the following question most definitely needs to be asked: what effects has this had on people diagnosed with the disparate collection of diseases encapsulated under the cancer label? (Bell, 2014) What does this tell us about the nature of 'courage'? An emerging area of exploration for health researchers is how individuals make sense of their experience of depression and find ways to describe their changing sense of (gendered) self in the process of recovery (Cardano, 2010). Qualitative health researchers in a range of areas have also explored how patients or health consumers use a wide range of metaphorical expressions when articulating and constructing their experiences of illness, distress and disease (Aita et al., 2003; Hall, 2011). In a recent analysis, Fullagar and O'Brien (2012) identified three key metaphors that women drew on to construct narratives about their 'recovering identities': the immobilising effects of depression, recovery as a battle to control depression, and recovery as a journey of feeling alive. The pervasiveness of media in all of everyday life has led to the notion that the way we experience our lives is mediated (Altheide, 2002).

Moral residue

We introduced moral residue first in Chapter 1.

It is widely conceded that, once an event that causes moral distress is over, the healthcare professional does not go back to his or her moral baseline afterwards. This is called 'moral residue', and refers to the fact that each time a morally distressing situation occurs and resolves, the level of residual moral distress continues to rise (Webster and Bayliss, 2000). Another way of looking at this concept is that moral distress can linger and, unfortunately, even grow with time (i.e. a 'moral residue crescendo'), with rather devastating long-term consequences. Two of the most serious problems are (1) becoming morally numb to ethically challenging situations and (2) developing clinician burnout and potentially leaving the profession (Hamric and Blackhall, 2007). Such serious risks remind us that moral distress is not benign; it behoves organisations to do what they can to prevent and snuff out moral distress as part of their strategic retention plan for employees.

A courage to practise

Medical training equips junior doctors with the courage to deal with distressing and difficult situations, arguably. In her excellent book, Rachel Clarke (2017: 67) opines that:

> Two experiences during my five years of medical school did more to shape how I would subsequently practise medicine than anything acquired from a textbook. This was the first. It took a brush with disaster to taste how disaster really feels. I now knew how little I grasped about the impact upon patients and relatives of the diagnoses of cancer I would one day deliver, of the news that I would break that a loved one had died, of the destruction I would come to unleash in my daily work as a doctor. There were whole realms of pain and fear about which I knew nothing and never would, unless I lived something like them. I vowed never to forget that.

The practice of medicine undoubtedly commands much courage – and an ever-frequent question for doctors has become: are the risks of practising 'worth it'? At the other extreme, some patients think doctors need to see their role in less heroic, arrogant terms but with much more humility. But what should we think when a medical professional makes a mistake?

> Medical mistakes are the stuff of nightmares: operating on the wrong limb; bad drug reactions; instruments left behind. But they're all too often an unfortunate reality. Reports suggest more than 250,000 people die per year due to medical errors, while millions more are harmed by drug-related mistakes. (Hughes, 2017)

The recent Bawa Garba case and the reaction of the GMC raise profound questions about organisational learning and regulation, particularly in relation to the 'blame culture' (e.g. www.bmj.com/content/359/bmj.j5534). We return to this specific case in Chapter 6.

There is possibly a long list of wider systemic factors that threaten a professional's ability to practise safely, beyond the direct control of that particular professional. Hospital staffing levels have recently been highlighted as a key ingredient for a safe care environment. Staffing levels have always been an issue for healthcare staff. 'What is the optimal level and mix of nursing staff required to deliver quality care as cost-effectively as possible?' is a continual question (see, for example: www.rcn.org.uk/get-help/rcn-advice/staffing-levels).

In recent times, concerns were founded on observations of poor care delivered by overstretched staff as part of the Mid Staffordshire NHS Foundation Trust

Public Inquiry (Department of Health, 2013b). Recommendations from the Francis report and the subsequent review by Don Berwick for the Department of Health into patient safety in the NHS have led to a renewed debate about safe staffing levels (Department of Health, 2013a). The National Institute for Health and Care Excellence (NICE) had commissioned the development of guidelines for safe levels of staffing (NICE 2014). The government then suspended NICE from producing further guidance on safe staffing levels in the NHS and this is a cause of great concern (see www.safestaffing.org.uk).

Healthcare is a safety-critical activity or, put another way, a quintessentially 'risky business', but this traditionally has not been very easily quantified. There is a critical need for reliable, robust research in this area. Despite the generation of mass data by the workforce, determining the impact of the contribution to patient safety remains challenging. Ensuring appropriate staffing and working hours is important to improve the quality and safety of care and to reduce care left undone in hospitals (Cho et al., 2016). Several cross-sectional studies have indicated a relationship between staffing and safety (Leary et al., 2017). This makes the building of predictive staffing models a challenge. Indeed, some sort of relationship between staffing and outcomes appears to exist. It appears to be non-linear but calculable, and a data-driven approach might be possible. An empirical mathematical model does need to be developed in wider policy terms (Leary et al., 2016). Variation in post-operative mortality rates has been associated with differences in registered nurse staffing levels. When nurse staffing levels are lower, there is also a higher incidence of necessary but missed nursing care. Ball and colleagues (2018) found that 'missed nursing care', which is highly related to nurse staffing, is associated with increased odds of patients dying in hospital following common surgical procedures. Such analyses support the hypothesis that missed nursing care mediates the relationship between registered nurse staffing and risk of patient mortality.

As an underpinning of high quality of care, patient safety has received increased attention as a growing body of evidence shows that medical errors, as a leading cause of death and injury, frequently occur worldwide in hospitals (Kohn et al., 2000). Patient safety involves constant surveillance of patients' conditions to prevent adverse events and early detection of patient deterioration (Clarke and Donaldson, 2008). Recio-Saucedo and colleagues (2015) recently searched ten electronic databases and relevant websites for English language studies published from 1994. Studies included reported a direct measure of nurse staffing relative to an activity measure (e.g. attendances, patient throughput) or an estimate of nurse staffing requirements. Randomised or non-randomised trials, prospective or retrospective observational, cross-sectional or correlational studies, interrupted time-series, and controlled before and after studies were all considered. The overall evidence was judged to be 'weak' but indicated that levels of nurse staffing in the emergency department are associated with patients leaving without being seen, emergency department care time and patient satisfaction. Intuitively, it appears rational to conclude that lower staffing levels and a decreased skill mix lead to a worsened patient experience, howeverso defined. But there is plenty more to do, across all settings, including inpatients and outpatients.

Human factors

See Chapter 3 for discussion of the profound impact of the inspirational work by Martin Bromiley, who founded the Clinical Human Factors Group.

Human factors research has identified what a positive safety culture looks and feels like (Dekker, 2007; Reason, 2000). In an open culture, staff feel comfortable discussing patient safety incidents and raising safety issues with both colleagues and senior managers, and in a 'just culture', staff, patients and carers are treated fairly, with empathy and consideration when they have been involved in a patient safety incident or have raised a safety issue. Every day in the NHS, tens of thousands of patients are treated safely by dedicated healthcare professionals who are motivated to provide high quality and safe clinical care. For the vast majority of patients, the treatment they receive alleviates or improves their symptoms, and is mostly a positive experience. However, an unacceptable number of patients are harmed as a result of their treatment or as a consequence of their admission to hospital. 'It is very rare for staff in healthcare to go to work with the intention of causing harm or failing to do the right thing. Therefore we have to ask why there are many incidents where some of the latent conditions are caused by staff not doing the right thing, even when they know what the right thing is' (Carthey and Clarke, 2010).

So are clinicians being 'courageous' by merely turning up to work? The answer to this lies in the severity of penalty if something unfortunately goes wrong. A doctor who makes a 'bad enough' medical error to cause the death of a patient can be prosecuted for criminal negligence manslaughter, but prosecutions were actually quite rare until the 1990s. With cases previously, the numbers of doctors charged had increased during the period 1990–2005, although few were convicted (McDowell and Ferner, 2013). Problems have arisen in the discussion of the jurisprudence of medical manslaughter as pointed out here:

> Just to turn for a moment then to the current test of liability, or the four limbs to this area of law: the duty of care; a breach of that duty, which causes, or significantly contributes, to the death of the victim; and then, crucially, those cases will hinge on whether that breach was so bad that it should be judged criminal.

This is a paraphrasing of the test from the leading case of Adomako, the House of Lords decision in 1995, where Lord Mackay, giving the only judgment in the case, provided the leading common law definition of gross negligence. Now, he acknowledged in his judgment that this test was circular, that if the jury asked (and juries often do ask) 'How negligent must the defendant have been so as to be criminal?' the correct answer is 'So negligent as to deserve a conviction for manslaughter'. So clearly there is an element of circularity to this test. However, it has survived numerous challenges through these cases (Quick, 2017).

The field is clearly 'work in progress'. It has now been announced that the General Medical Council's independent review to explore how cases of gross negligence manslaughter and culpable homicide (in Scotland) are initiated and investigated in the UK, and how these apply to medical practice, will be led by Dame Clare Marx (www.gmc-uk.org/news/media-centre/media-centre-archive/dame-clare-marx-to-lead-medical-manslaughter-review). In 2014, it was reported that a consultant urologist who was jailed for manslaughter after he failed to treat a life-threatening infection in a young mother quickly enough had been allowed to return to work under conditions set by a fitness-to-practise panel (Dyer, 2014).

It might be that courage is required to practise under such circumstances with compassion and courage. The close association between competence, compassion and courage is detailed here:

> Compassionate clinical practice guidelines for healthcare providers for respectful disposition after miscarriage are presented. When woven into the whole of a clinician's practice, these guidelines provide the framework for giving women and their families the care they want and deserve when experiencing miscarriage. Relying on theoretical concepts of personhood, place, and protection, care providers can assess the unique meaning a woman assigns to her early pregnancy loss and offer interventions that embrace the concept of respectful disposition. Respectful methods of disposition involve a continuum of care that shows respect for remains and relies on person-, family-, and culture-centered nursing care. Policies, practices, and perspectives that flow from respectful disposition have women and families at their core and flexibility to co-create care. This involves courage and competence. (Levang et al., 2018: 19)

We will come back to 'human factors' again in Chapter 5.

Courage and the 'patient experience'

Practitioners and professionals are not the only ones who need 'courage' – patients and service users need lots of courage too, often unspoken of in their daily interactions, but certainly much reflected upon. Furthermore, there has been a skew in thinking about 'reflective practice' in the context of health and social care to concentrate on issues such as postoperative complications, missed diagnosis, or a patient with any sort of grievance, but equally valuable are accounts of patient experiences which make sense of any given situation (e.g. Koshy et al., 2017).

Previous research by Haase (1987) relating to courage had addressed the manner of courage development in chronically ill adolescents with a variety of illnesses. Haase concluded that asking patients to be brave should be avoided, because in her study participants described the presence of courage as 'coming and going'. Furthermore, Deborah Finfgeld took this forward, and over a number of years conducted a programme of research devoted to courage, investigating it in the chronically ill elderly and in middle-aged adults and young adults with long-term health concerns. She, interestingly, concluded that courage develops over time and includes fully accepting reality, problem solving and the need to push beyond on-going struggles (reviewed in Donohue-Porter, 2013).

Finfgeld (1999: 803) specifically notes:

> Courageous behavior is characterized by efforts to be productive, make contributions, and help others and results in a sense of personal integrity and thriving. Courage is promoted and sustained by several interrelated intrapersonal and interpersonal forces as well as the reflective awareness that one has developed a courageous persona.

Surgery

Many research participants have previous negative experiences of surgery, for example complications, severe nausea and vomiting, or uncaring encounters with staff, which increased their anxiety. Preparing oneself therefore meant finding courage in an unfamiliar and highly technical environment, despite anxiety and even panic. In this phase, the expected loss of control was mastered as was anxiety about what would happen: 'You are at the mercy of other people who literally have your life in their hands. I can't check or know what they are doing but I trust they are doing the right things and that all will be well' (Liebenhagen and Forsberg, 2013: 276).

Diabetes

A purpose of a recent study was to explore the experience of nurses in relation to courage development in patients with disabling complications of diabetes (Donohue-Porter, 2013).

This qualitative study used phenomenological inquiry and included face-to-face interviews of nurses to explore their experience in assisting patients in the development of courage. The experience of courage is investigated as it relates to a specific group of patients who have complications of diabetes. Four categories representing the unique opportunities for courage development by nurses were generated. These categories included education, advocacy, relationship building and humanisation. Each category described nursing intentions and actions and taken together formed an essential structure of courage development. The study concluded that nurses recognise and are able to describe their role in courage development. Implications for improved health through deliberate caring nursing interventions, aimed at courage development, are presented.

Courage and 'living'

An article by Christensen and Mikkelsen (2008) addressed the complexity of children's risk landscapes through an ethnography of 10- to 12-year-old Danish children. The data revealed how children individually and collectively engaged with risk in their everyday activities. The children assessed risks in relation to their perceptions of their health as strength and control, negotiated the conditions of playing, and attuned their responses to situations of potential social and physical conflict. Examples were given by the authors of positive risk engagement illustrated in a variety of contexts: children's decisions to wear or not to wear a bicycle helmet; playing and games and routine pushing and shoving at school. In looking after themselves, children negotiate rules of participation and they safeguard personal and collective interests. The authors argued that risk engagement is an important resource through which children also learn from their own mistakes. This is a necessary learning process when children engage with their personal health and safety. This is an example of courage needed to embrace living with risk to improve health.

In Harper Lee's well-known novel *To Kill a Mockingbird*, the protagonist Atticus Finch tells his children, 'I wanted you to see what real courage is, instead of getting the idea that courage is a man with a gun in his hand. It's when you know you're licked before you begin, but you begin anyway and see it through no matter what' (cited in McCartney, 2014).

Some patients show amazing courage (Wilkinson, 2016) in dealing with medical conditions, and can indeed be a significant source of inspiration to others facing similar situations:

> The damage to the soft tissues of her pelvis was profound. Despite numerous and varied attempts at surgical cure, she had recurrence of her fistulas and continued to experience constant leaking of urine and stool. One year in the hospital, and with no hope in sight, she had regained an ever-present smile and sense of humour that belied her wretched state. She helped with the teaching and care of the other fistula patients and became a source of inspiration for patients and staff alike. (p. 1393)

In day-to-day life, courage may be essential for wellbeing and resilience. One way of trying to comprehend the mental health status of Aboriginal people in Kempsey is to consider how precisely they deal with social injustices, high morbidity and mortality rates, substance abuse, domestic violence and unemployment. The standard 'bio-psycho-social model' may not be the most suitable framework to understand the Aboriginal notions of emotional health and wellbeing. The approach also seems unable to cope with the intricacies of the remarkable resilience of particular Aboriginal communities or individuals, although there are found to be many examples of strength and courage in the face of trauma, death and discrimination (Cleworth et al., 2006). It takes, however, a lot to be courageous about mortality. Atul Gawande's book on *Being Mortal* (2015: 9) explores sensitively the issues:

> This is a book about the modern experience of mortality – about what it's like to be creatures who age and die, how medicine has changed the experience and how it hasn't, where our ideas about how to deal with our finitude have got the reality wrong.

Four years ago, Barbara Ehrenreich, 76, reached the realisation that she was old enough to die. She had undergone a myriad of preventive medical tests or restricting her diet in pursuit of a longer life. The experience of cancer treatment helped shape her thoughts on ageing, she says:

> Within this last decade, I realised I was not going to go through chemotherapy again. That's like a year out of your life when you consider the recovery time and everything. I don't have a year to spare. (quoted in Rock, 2018)

In her new book *Natural Causes*, Ehrenreich (2018) writes about how you receive more calls to screenings and tests in the US – including mammograms, colonoscopies and bone density scans – as you get older. She claims most 'fail the evidence-based test' and are at best unnecessary and worst harmful.

Many patients themselves have faced spectacular personal battles, and quite often they will not speak to others about them. Linda Costigan struggled to quit smoking. She was finally successful – but only after she had been diagnosed with lung cancer. By then she had been smoking for 42 years. Although her own prognosis was poor, Costigan tried to do what she could to educate others about the hazards of smoking (Haviland et al., 2003). But the plethora of reasons explaining an individual's personal reaction to a condition remains unclear. Religion, for example, plays a critical role in the process through which individual patients confront diseases, enabling patients to find meaning in life or develop a sense of belonging (Tsai et al., 2016). According to Koenig (2012), religion positively influences spiritual, emotional and mental health.

Facing up to severe illness cannot be underestimated by people who have never had this particular experience. Tremors, stiffness and slowness of movement led a 35-year-old woman to consult her family practitioner. The much feared and not welcomed diagnosis was early onset Parkinson's disease. Meeting a family physician with whom she can jointly manage the disease, arguably, however, has given this patient courage to face the future (Hayes, 1994: 507):

> When the diagnosis was confirmed and the shock had worn off for those close to me, it was back to business as usual. After all, they assumed, the medication controlled the symptoms, and being a usually optimistic person, I gave the illusion of having everything under control. Friends and

family assumed that everything was back to normal, and I was coping just fine, thank you.

Actually this couldn't have been further from the truth. I was in turmoil. What about my family? My future? Will I ever meet a man who will love me enough to be able to take my unpredictable future in stride? What made things worse was that I had no empathetic professional to talk with. The neurology clinic I attend is renowned for its expertise, but I'm just a number. Basically I don't like going there. The waiting room is always full of patients in very advanced stages of Parkinson's. I find that scary. Besides it's an hour's drive away, and appointments are now being made 2 months in advance. (Hayes, 1994: 507)

How people actually react to a serious diagnosis is a critical issue for health and social care professionals, and surprisingly relatively under-investigated. Kate Swaffer, a leading advocate for people living with dementia, herself living with dementia, notes the following in her celebrated memoir, *What the Hell Happened to my Brain?* (2016: 41):

I have said this previously, but the diagnosis of dementia really did feel like a pseudo-death, of me, of who I am, my history, and then the fear of who I might become.

The first few weeks I cried non-stop, tears that felt as if they would never go away. Together, my husband and I walked almost every day for exercise and leisure, and some of those days, I started running, with salty tears running down my blotchy cheeks like river torrents. I cried and cried and cried, and thought they would never stop, but after you run long enough, the pain takes over and gives you something else to think about! It worked, at least when I was running.

You can also need the courage to face medical treatment. And this can be at a very basic level. It is not unusual for a patient to fear the needles used for phlebotomy, intravenous line insertions, subcutaneous or intramuscular injections, needle aspirations, and even those needles used to inject something to eliminate pain (local anaesthetics). The origins of the fear may be multiple and range from a previous bad experience to being threatened with getting a shot for bad behaviour as a child (Goodspeed and Lee, 2011).

Courage can also be needed with more complex therapy. Studies have progressively shown that a number of women do not receive adjuvant radiation therapy following breast-conserving surgery; the reasons have not been well investigated. Recently, in a groundbreaking study (Guidolin et al., 2018), the charts of 267 patients who did not receive radiation therapy following surgery, in order to determine patient-stated reasons for non-receipt, were reviewed. It was found that 43% of patients did not receive radiation because they received a completion mastectomy. Excluding these patients, reasons for non-receipt of radiation therapy were sorted into categories. Most patients declined radiation therapy (against physician advice). Guidolin and colleagues (2018) identified three major barriers to receipt of radiation therapy: improper patient selection, transportation or ambulatory issues and patient fear surrounding radiation toxicity.

Coming to terms with any condition which impacts on your living demands a whole person perspective, and courage is critically at the centre of the emotional responses of very many patients and service users. Clinical guideline suggestions for health professionals working with families of children or adolescents diagnosed with cancer within the first year following the diagnosis have been scrutinised. Health professionals must listen to and accept the emotions of shock, anger and loss by the family members who are facing the potential loss of their healthy child together with the upheaval in their lives and disruptions to their plans for the future. Health professionals should be encouraged to provide clear information to the whole family in relation to the treatment plan and caring strategies for the child (Mu et al., 2015). Encouraging the family members of children with cancer to develop positive thinking and to plan for their future life should be a priority of the nursing care plan.

Psychologists and psychotherapists working with people experiencing different difficulties are used to helping people to understand their experiences of an 'existential crisis' and can often help other professionals, patients and families to understand this normal response to illness. A perspective of existential crisis is presented through special experiences requiring explanation of meaning and purpose. The attempt is made to present a holistic understanding of existential crisis, differentiating the main components and aspects of existential crisis (Butėnaitė et al., 2016). It has been previously noted that despair and helplessness are also aspects of an existential crisis. In the present moment, a person is experiencing a struggle of opposites between freedom and dependence, which causes inner-pervasive despair (Kierkegaard, 1941). The attempt to deny one's own individuality and avoid the anxiety of non-existence causes despair and emptiness in a person's life (May, 1977).

Courage to inspire

Clinicians are often patients themselves too. Kate Granger trained at Edinburgh University, graduating with honours in 2005. She was eventually told she was suffering desmoplastic small round cell tumour. This aggressive form of cancer affects just one in two million people, usually children and teenagers. She said she wanted healthcare professionals to understand what being a patient was really like. Despite having to cope with constant ill-health and the effects of treatment, Dr Granger remained dedicated to her work. During her visits to hospital as a patient, she was unimpressed that so few healthcare workers introduced themselves, so she decided to start the #hellomynameis campaign. The idea was to reinforce the valuable nature of introductions and to ask people throughout the care sector to pledge their commitment to introducing themselves properly to each patient they meet. Kate Granger wrote in *The Guardian* on 2 February 2015:

> As a patient, you are in a vulnerable position. The healthcare team knows so much personal information about you, yet you often know nothing about them. This results in a very one-sided power imbalance. A simple introduction can help to redress this imbalance. I also believe it is the first rung on the ladder to providing compassionate care by establishing a human connection and building trust with a person.

Courage and 'life events' including death

On 19 February 2015, Oliver Sacks published in the *New York Times*:

> A month ago, I felt that I was in good health, even robust health. At 81, I still swim a mile a day. But my luck has run out — a few weeks ago I learned that I have multiple metastases in the liver. Nine years ago it was discovered that I had a rare tumor of the eye, an ocular melanoma. The radiation and lasering to remove the tumor ultimately left me blind in that eye. But though ocular melanomas metastasize in perhaps 50 percent of cases, given the particulars of my own case, the likelihood was much smaller. I am among the unlucky ones. I feel grateful that I have been granted nine years of good health and productivity since the original diagnosis, but now I am face to face with dying. The cancer occupies a third of my liver, and though its advance may be slowed, this particular sort of cancer cannot be halted.

Sacks cited David Hume, who, upon learning that he was mortally ill at age 65, wrote a short autobiography in a single day in April of 1776. David Hume (born 1711) was a Scottish philosopher, historian, economist and essayist, who is best known today for his highly influential system of philosophical empiricism, scepticism and naturalism. Sacks titled it *My Own Life*. 'I now reckon upon a speedy dissolution', he wrote. 'I have suffered very little pain from my disorder; and what is more strange, have, notwithstanding the great decline of my person, never suffered a moment's abatement of my spirits. I possess the same ardour as ever in study, and the same gaiety in company.' Oliver Sacks later died on 30 August 2015.

Courage may be shown in the bravery of moving into a nursing home (Anderson, 2016). Jim Anderson writes:

> When she first moved to a nursing home, she was really upset at the beginning, but in a matter of days she showed the spark that led her through a life full of social graces. I went to visit her soon after she had

moved in to the nursing home, and was invited to join her for a meal in facilities dining room... The same Jim Anderson who had brought her here just a day or two earlier, much to her chagrin. To have such grace and forgiveness in such circumstances reflected an immense amount of bravery.

Courageous leaders in end-of-life care can focus on four leadership qualities: (*a*) best care for patients and their families, (*b*) best care for the nursing and other staff who care for patients at the end of life, (*c*) developing systems that support the best care in end-of-life situations in our organisations, and (*d*) our communities and nation. It will take the courage of leaders to advocate for implementing known evidence in the face of many obstacles within the healthcare system (Kerfoot, 2012). Seriously ill patients tend to adjust their life goals, hopes and the way they want to live and experience their new life in accordance with the new situation (Rohde et al., 2017).

Being with dying people is an integral part of healthcare yet many staff feel unprepared to accompany people through the process of dying, reporting a lack of skills in psychosocial and spiritual care, resulting in high levels of moral distress, grief and burnout. 'Just being there' with a patient involves personal courage, especially when they are caring for desolate and despairing patients. Facing patients' suffering may open the nurses' own wounds and trigger feelings of helplessness, vulnerability and uncertainty (Tornøe et al., 2014: 7). Family members move to incorporate loss into their lives, and to shift to new, changed, but continuing relationships (Moules et al., 2007). The nature of these conversations of suffering (Wright, 2005) in grief might be seen as spiritual conversations, and the willingness to enter them requires a degree of courage on the part of the practitioner, as well as a veneration of the sacredness, privilege and healing possibilities of such conversations.

Crying has been studied from the perspective of family members of patients in palliative care. The aim of a recent day study was to explore the significance of family members crying in a palliative care context with special reference to factors that influence crying. Interviews were carried out with 14 family members of patients admitted to palliative care (Rydé et al., 2008). Family members felt that in normal cases, crying was a very private part of themselves. It was not possible to start crying anywhere or anyhow. First, certain conditions had to be fulfilled. One of the conditions for crying was the attitude to crying. Their personal history and childhood as well as their sex influenced their own crying attitude and could be either approving or disapproving. Even in death, it is possible to demonstrate courage. It is not known how widespread a practice it is for mourners to write and deliver a eulogy at a funeral, and it may be that correspondents commented on it precisely because it is unusual. Indeed, speakers would hardly be praised for their courage in speaking if such speeches were routine (Bailey and Walter, 2016). Making sense of a death can be a fruitful exercise.

Facing up to mortality and dying, and courage, needs very little explanation, but accounts are still remarkably informative and instructive.

Sharon Kendall (2006) details one of the findings of a large phenomenological study into the effects of nurse–patient encounters on clinical learning and practice. Every nurse faces the challenge of caring for a patient with cancer at some point in his or her nursing career. The participants, 392 nurses, were asked to provide an account of a care episode from their practice. These narrative/clinical exemplars were for a patient with a diagnosis of cancer and participants were asked to discuss the impact this encounter had on clinical learning and clinical practice. Each day nurses occasionally encounter a person who inspires them, someone they admire because of their courage. Responses from the participants identified a number of such people. Nurses used 'powerful language, brave, strong, courageous, to describe these patients'. The diagnosis of cancer is undoubtedly a daunting prospect and is seen as a challenge physically and emotionally.

Consoling existential and spiritual distress is a deeply personal and relational practice. Nurses have a potential to alleviate existential and spiritual suffering through a consoling presence. By connecting deeply with patients and their families, nurses have the possibility to affirm the patients' strength and facilitate their courage to live a meaningful life and die a dignified death (Tornøe et al., 2014: 7):

> Our results show that becoming willing and ready to 'just be there', seeing and listening to the wounded patient demanded personal courage, especially when they were caring for desolate and despairing patients. Facing patients' suffering could sometimes open the nurses' own wounds and trigger feelings of helplessness, vulnerability, and uncertainty. The nurses expressed that giving and receiving peer support and debriefing was vital to endure the emotional pressures of being with the dying.

Being with dying people is an integral part of nursing, yet many nurses feel unprepared to accompany people through the process of dying (Rushton et al., 2007). Listening and staying present as the patients' suffering unfolds can be emotionally challenging because it exposes the nurses to their own vulnerability and finitude (Cody, 2007; Naef, 2006).

And understanding how grieving family members cope is now to be welcomed, rather than simply dismissed as unimportant. Joshua Titcombe, James' son, had died two and a half years earlier because of poor care in the 24 hours after his birth at Furness General Hospital in Cumbria. James Titcombe (2017) comments:

> Signs that he was suffering from a serious infection that should have resulted in speedy medical referral were not acted on by the midwives looking after him. Instead, Joshua's first contact with a doctor came some 24 hours later when his mother found him collapsed in his cot and called for help. By this time, however, it was too late. Despite being transferred to two different neonatal intensive care units and putting up a fight to be proud of, Joshua died eight days later ... Joshua's brief time in this world was as medicalised as any experience of maternity care could be, yet his dire predicament could have been avoided with the simplest and cheapest of medical interventions.

And it is one thing coping with living and dying, but it is an altogether another thing when you find yourself having to muster up courage over your son's death as well as the failings in the NHS. Titcombe (2015: 172) commented previously:

> It is one thing when you find out your local hospital has suffered serious failings in care resulting in numerous preventable deaths, it is another when you find that hospital is involved, if not in blatant cover-up, in obscuring the extent of the problems. But when you find the organisations responsible for regulating hospitals have not only failed to maintain stand-ards but are complicit in their own cover-ups then you can begin to despair whether you will ever get to the bottom of just how and why these trag-edies occurred. This was the picture that began to emerge in 2013.

Finally, dying from cancer tends to be seen as 'painful', 'dragging on' and causing extreme suffering, while dying from heart disease is seen as 'quick and neat', 'natural' and 'relatively painless' (Davison et al., 1991; Emslie et al., 2001). What constitutes a good death has been well researched, and various common characteristics of 'a good death' have been reported across studies (Hales et al., 2010; Kehl, 2006). Examples of these include, perhaps, being comfortable (i.e. with adequate control of pain and other symptoms) and being afforded dignity and privacy (Emanuel and Emanuel, 1998; Smith, 2000).

Depression

Accounts of life-changing events always remind a healthcare professional that it is a unique privilege to care for any patient or 'service user'. Such narratives invari-ably disclose deeply personal responses to personal events, including the disclosure of a diagnosis or shortcomings of treatment or communication. They remind the reader that much of medicine and nursing is not contained within the pages of a textbook. They also serve as a caution to all of us of the frailty and vulnerability of the human condition, and that many people, despite outward experiences, are actually very scared. Courage is therefore an integral part of living, and necessary to 'live better'.

Professor Linda Gask spent more than 30 years working as a psychiatrist despite personally experiencing recurring periods of anxiety and depression. She eventu-ally became a professor of psychiatry at the University of Manchester, has been an advisor to the World Health Organisation, and trained health professionals in many different countries in how to listen and talk to people with mental health problems. She is passionate about reaching a wider audience in order to bust the stigma that continues to prevent people from getting the help they really need.

The Other Side of Silence (2015: 9) is her highly acclaimed memoir weaving her own experience with that of her patients, while giving an insight into some of the therapeutic answers for people suffering from depression. Her book shows it is possible to experience depression, but still have a happy life and build a career. But she describes brilliantly the crippling nature of depression:

> The problem is that when you are caught deep in the jaws of depression, recapturing a sense of hope seems almost unimaginable. Low mood colours the ways in which we see our lives and clouds our judgement, not only about others but most importantly about ourselves. It is hard to think positively, as others insist, when you consider yourself to be completely worthless.

She emphasises the importance of both biological and psychosocial factors in the origins of this illness and her description of treatments is both fair and accurate (Brown, 2017). Gask (2015: 40–41) describes some of her own experiences:

> There came a point when I couldn't go on. My head was splitting open and I struggled to hold the pieces of my brain together. I can't remember exactly what happened. I was sitting in the flat, obsessing over the timetable and my failure to comply with it, while at the time listening so intently to the noise of the people in the tenement stairwell. They were walking up and down and chatting to each other about the weather and whose it turn it was to clean the stairs, as though everything was quite normal. I was acutely aware of the sounds of the main door on the street clanging shut ... I wasn't sleeping or working, just sobbing.

Courage and careers in health and social care

Someone who struggled through childhood in the home of a parent who has suffered from an active alcoholic dependence syndrome may need to be very brave to respond not only with technical competence but also with respect and empathy to an alcoholic patient in liver failure on his ward. As one of the authors of this book, I am living in recovery from alcoholism, succeeding in not having had a drink for 11 continuous years at the time of submission of this manuscript. Such a 'wounded healer' may still be living with considerable emotional wounds. We cannot exactly know the courage it takes for any nurse or physician or therapist to approach, much less to give attentive and compassionate care to, a patient who is the embodiment of his or her unresolved grief (Hamric et al., 2015).

Arguably, a different sort of courage is needed to do something brand new and very risky at the outset. It has been more than 50 years since Dr Christiaan Barnard, a South African cardiac surgeon together with his multidisciplinary team, successfully performed the world's first human-to-human heart transplantation at the Groote Schuur Hospital in Cape Town, South Africa. On 3 December 1967, Lewis Washkansky, suffering from severe heart failure at the age of 53, received the heart of 25-year-old Denise Darvall, who tragically died in a car accident. Following this revolutionary operation, Dr Barnard became a celebrity virtually overnight. And indeed, it was the beginning of a long journey during the next 50 years which was driven by courage, innovation and, importantly, persistence (Emmert, 2017).

A certain degree of courage is needed in career development. Recent studies have begun to examine the role of behavioural courage in career-related outcomes, suggesting that courageous behaviours influence positive work behavioural outcomes, personal identity and prosocial behaviours (e.g. Howard et al., 2016; Koerner, 2014). Additionally, it has been found that adolescents with high levels of courage are likely more motivated to reach their plans and to think about and implement different solutions for achieving them, have more coping skills to achieve them, reducing the feeling of fear (Ginevra and Capozza, 2015; Magnano et al. 2017). Central to the life design paradigm is the concept of career adaptability, that is an essential resource to help individuals plan their uncertain future, face adverse working conditions, adapt to changes in the job market and job conditions, and therefore increase their wellbeing (Savickas, 2015). In this current socio-economic context, particular relevance is also given to the propensity of individuals to behave courageously and persist despite perceived risks (behavioural courage), as this resource seems to be a strength when making difficult career choices despite fears related to the future, and a resource related to personal wellbeing (Ginevra et al., 2018).

For a few, medical science is a true vocation rather than simply a 'career choice'. Darwin's theories of evolution and natural selection are intrinsically dwarfed by the courage, persistence and risk-taking required to implement such thinking.

Useful Weblinks

www.yorkshireeveningpost.co.uk/news/kate-granger-yorkshire-doctor-who-inspired-the-world-1-8030893
www.theguardian.com/healthcare-network/2014/may/21/friendly-introduction-transform-patient-experience
www.theguardian.com/commentisfree/2017/aug/14/royal-college-midwives-normal-birth-joshua-titcombe

References

Aita, V., McIlvain, H., Susman, J. and Crabtree, B. (2003) 'Using metaphor as a qualitative analytic approach to understand complexity in primary care research', *Qualitative Health Research*, *13*: 1419–1431.

Altheide, D. (2002) *Creating Fear: News and the Construction of Crisis*. Hawthorne, NY: Aldine de Gruyter.

Anderson, J. (2016) 'The bravery of people with dementia', *Clinical Advisor*, 20 April. Available at: www.clinicaladvisor.com/the-waiting-room/the-bravery-of-dementia-patients/article/491112 (accessed 5 June 2018).

Bailey, T. and Walter, T. (2016) 'Funerals against death', *Mortality*, 21(2): 149–166.

Ball, J.E., Bruyneel, L., Aiken, L.H., Sermeus, W., Sloane, D.M., Rafferty, A..M, Lindqvist, R., Tishelman, C. and Griffiths, P. (2018) 'Post-operative mortality, missed care and nurse staffing in nine countries: A cross-sectional study', *International Journal of Nursing Studies*, 78: 10–15.

Beach, W.A., Easter, D.W., Good, J.S. and Pigeron, E. (2005) 'Disclosing and responding to cancer "fears" during oncology interviews', *Social Science & Medicine*, 60: 893–910.

Bell, K. (2014) 'The breast-cancer-ization of cancer survivorship: Implications for experiences of the disease', *Social Science and Medicine*, 110: 56–63.

Brown, T. (2017) 'Review- *The Other Side of Silence: A Psychiatrist's Memoir of Depression*', *BJPsych Bulletin*, 41(2): 125.

Butėnaitė, J., Bulotaitė, L. and Mockus, A (2016) 'Components of existential crisis: A theoretical analysis', *International Journal of Psychology: Biopsychosocial Approach*, 18: 9–27.

Cardano, M. (2010) 'Mental distress: Strategies of sense-making', *Health*, 14(3): 253–271.

Carthey, J. and Clarke, J. (2010) *Implementing Human Factors in Healthcare, a Patient Safety First guide*. Available at: www.weahsn.net/wp-content/uploads/Human-Factors-How-to-Guide-v1.2.pdf (accessed 5 June 2018).

Cho, E., Lee, N.J., Kim, E.Y., Kim, S., Lee, K., Park, K.O. and Sung, Y.H. (2016) 'Nurse staffing level and overtime associated with patient safety, quality of care, and care left undone in hospitals: A cross-sectional study', *International Journal of Nursing Studies*, 60: 263–271.

Christensen, P. and Mikkelsen, M.R. (2008) 'Jumping off and being careful: Children's strategies of risk management in everyday life', Sociology of Health & Illness, 30(1): 112–130.

Clarke, J.N. (1992) 'Cancer, heart disease and AIDS: What do the media tell us about these diseases?', *Health Communication*, 4(2): 105–120.

Clarke, R. (2017) *Your Life in my Hands*. London: Metro Books.

Clarke, S.P. and Donaldson, N.E. (2008) 'Nurse staffing and patient care quality and safety identifying nurse sensitive outcomes', in *Patient Safety and Quality: An Evidence-Based Handbook for Nurses*. Rockville, MD: Agency for Healthcare Research and Quality. pp. 111–136.

Cleworth, S., Smith, W. and Sealey, R. (2006) 'Grief and courage in a river town: A pilot project in the Aboriginal community of Kempsey, New South Wales', *Australas Psychiatry*, 14(4): 390–394.

Cody, W. (2007) 'Bearing witness to suffering: Participating in cotranscendence', *International Journal of Human Caring*, 11(2): 17.

Davison, C., Smith, G.D. and Frankel, S. (1991) 'Lay epidemiology and the prevention paradox: The implications of coronary candidacy for health education', *Sociology of Health and Illness*, 13(1): 1–19.

Dekker, S. (2007) *Just Culture Balancing Safety and Accountability*. London: Ashgate Publishing Company.

Department of Health (2013a) *Berwick Review into Patient Safety*. London: Department of Health.

Department of Health (2013b) *Report of the Mid Staffordshire NHS Foundation Trust Public Inquiry*. London: Department of Health. Available at: www.midstaffspublicinquiry.com/report (accessed 5 June 2018).

Donohue-Porter, P. (2013) 'Nursing's role in courage development in patients facing complications of diabetes', *Journal of Holistic Nursing*, 31(1): 49–61.

Dyer, C. (2014) 'Urologist who was jailed for manslaughter is allowed back to work', *BMJ*, 349: g4931.

Ehrenreich, B. (2010) Smile! You've got cancer, *The Guardian* (2 Jan 2010), https://www. theguardian.com/lifeandstyle/2010/jan/02/cancer-positive-thinkingbarbara-ehrenreich (online, accessed 13 Sep 2018).

Ehrenreich, B. (2018) *Natural Causes: An Epidemic of Wellness, the Certainty of Dying, and Killing Ourselves to Live Longer*. New York: Hachette Book Group.

Emanuel, E.J. and Emanuel, L.L. (1998) 'The promise of a good death', *Lancet, 351* (Supplement II): 21–29.

Emmert, M.Y. (2017) 'Fifty years of heart transplantation: A journey of courage, innovation and persistence, celebrated in Cape Town', *European Heart Journal, 38*(46): 3405.

Emslie, C., Hunt, K. and Watt, G. (2001) 'I'd rather go with a heart attack than drag on: Lay images of heart disease and the problems they present for primary and secondary prevention', *Coronary Health Care, 5*(1): 25–32.

Fife, B.L. and Wright, E.C. (2000) 'The dimensionality of stigma: A comparison of its impact on the self of persons with HIV/AIDS and cancer', *Journal of Health and Social Behaviour, 41*: 50–67.

Finfgeld, D.L. (1999) 'Courage as a process of pushing beyond the struggle', *Qualitative Health Research, 9*(6): 803–814.

Frankl, V. (1939) *Man's Search for Meaning*. New York, NY: Pocket Books.

Fullagar, S. and O'Brien, W. (2012) 'Immobility, battles, and the journey of feeling alive: Women's metaphors of self-transformation through depression and recovery', *Qualitative Health Research, 22*(8): 1063–1072.

Gask, L. (2015) *The Other Side of Silence*. Chichester, West Sussex: Summersdale Publishers.

Gawande, A. (2015) *Being Mortal*. London: Profile Books Ltd.

Ginevra, M.C. and Capozza, D. (2015) 'Il coraggio: Dalle definizioni ad alcune considerazioni per le attività di counselling [Courage: From definition to some suggestions for counselling activities]', in L. Nota and S. Soresi (eds), *Il counselling del futuro*. Padova, Italy: Cleup. pp. 111–122.

Ginevra, M.C., Magnano, P., Lodi, E., Annovazzi, C., Camussi, E., Patrizi, P. and Nota, L. (2018) 'The role of career adaptability and courage on life satisfaction in adolescence', *Journal of Adolescence, 62*: 1–8.

Goodspeed, R.B. and Lee, B.Y. (2011) 'What if … a patient is highly fearful of needles?', *Journal of Ambulatory Care Management, 34*(2): 203–204.

Gould, N.H. (2005) 'Courage: Its nature and development', *Journal of Humanistic Counseling Education and Development, 44*(1): 102–116.

Granger, K. (2015) 'I want my legacy to be that the NHS treats all patients with compassion', *The Guardian*, 'Views from the NHS frontline', https://www.theguardian.com/healthcarenetwork/ 2014/may/21/friendly-introduction-transform-patient-experience (online, accessed 13 Sep 2018).

Guidolin, K., Lock, M. and Brackstone, M. (2018) 'Patient-perceived barriers to radiation therapy for breast cancer', *Canadian Journal of Surgery, 61*(2): 141–143.

Haase, J. (1987) 'Components of courage in chronically ill adolescents: A phenomenological study', *Advances in Nursing Science, 9*(2): 64–80.

Hales, S., Zimmermann, C. and Rodin, G. (2010) 'Review: The quality of dying and death – A systematic review of measures', *Palliative Medicine, 24*(2): 127–144.

Hall, J.M. (2011) 'Narrative methods in a study of trauma recovery', *Qualitative Health Research, 21*: 3–13.

Hamric, A.B. and Blackhall, L.J. (2007) 'Nurse–physician perspectives on the care of dying patients in intensive care units: Collaboration, moral distress, and ethical climate', *Critical Care Medicine, 35*(2): 422–429.

Hamric, A.B., Arras, J.D. and Mohrmann, M.E. (2015) 'Must we be courageous?', *Hastings Center Report*, 45(3): 33–40.

Haviland, L., Healton, C.G., Fee, E., Brown, T.M., Toomey, B.A. and Kastens, B. (2003) 'Courage and dignity', *American Journal of Public Health*, 93(7): 1045.

Hayes, L. (1994) 'Early onset Parkinson's disease. Part 1: The patient's story', *Canadian Family Physician*, 40: 506–508.

Health Advisory Service (1982) *The Rising Tide: Developing Services for Mental Illness in Old Age*. London: HMSO.

Horwitz, A. and Wakefield, J. (2007) *The Loss of Sadness: How Psychiatry Transformed Normal Sorrow into Depressive Disorder*. New York: Oxford University Press.

Howard, M.C., Farr, J.L., Grandey, A.A. and Gutworth, M.B. (2016) 'The creation of the Workplace Social Courage Scale (WSCS): An investigation of internal consistency, psychometric properties, validity, and utility', *Journal of Business and Psychology*, 32: 1–18. Available at: http://dx.doi.org/10.1007/s10869-016-9463-8 (accessed 5 June 2018).

Hughes, L. (2017) 'How concerned should you be about medical errors?', *WebMD*. Available at: www.webmd.com/a-to-z-guides/features/medical-mistakes-what-you-should-know- (accessed 5 June 2018).

Johannessen, A., Engedal, K. and Thorsen, K. (2015) 'Adult children of parents with young-onset dementia narrate the experiences of their youth through metaphors', *The Journal of Multidisciplinary Healthcare*, 27(8): 245–254.

Kehl, K.A. (2006) 'Moving toward peace: An analysis of the concept of a good death', *American Journal of Hospice and Palliative Medicine*, 23(4): 277–286.

Kendall, S. (2006) 'Admiring courage: Nurses' perceptions of caring for patients with cancer', *European Journal of Oncology Nursing*, 10(5): 324–334.

Kennedy, J.F. (1955) *Profiles in Courage*. New York, NY: Harper & Row.

Kerfoot, K.M. (2012) 'Courage, leadership, and end-of-life care: When courage counts', *Nursing Economics*, 30(3): 176–178.

Kierkegaard, S. (1941) *The Sickness Unto Death*. Princeton, NJ: Princeton University Press.

Koenig, H.G. (2012) 'Religion, spirituality, and health: The research and clinical implications', *ISRN Psychiatry*: 278730.

Koerner, M. M. (2014) 'Courage as identity work: Accounts of workplace courage', *Academy of Management Journal*, 57(1): 63–93.

Kohn, L.T., Corrigan, J.M. and Donaldson, M.S. (2000) *To Err is Human: Building a Safer Health System*. Washington, DC: National Academies Press.

Koshy, K., Limb, C., Gundogan, B., Whitehurst, K. and Jafree, D.J. (2017) 'Reflective practice in health care and how to reflect effectively', *International journal of surgery*. Oncology, 2(6): e20.

Lane, H.P., McLachlan, S. and Philip, J. (2013) 'The war against dementia: Are we battle weary yet?', *Age Ageing*, 42(3): 281–283.

Leary, A., Cook, R., Jones, S., Smith, J., Gough, M., Maxwell, E., Punshon, G. and Radford, M. (2016) 'Mining routinely collected acute data to reveal non-linear relationships between nurse staffing levels and outcomes', *BMJ*, 6(12): e011177.

Leary, A., Tomai, B., Swift, A., Woodward, A. and Hurst, K. (2017) 'Nurse staffing levels and outcomes – mining the UK national data sets for insight', *International Journal of Health Care Quality Assurance*, 30(3): 235–247.

Levang, E., Limbo, R. and Ziegler, T.R. (2018) 'Respectful disposition after miscarriage: Clinical practice recommendations', *American Journal of Maternal/Child Nursing*, 43(1): 19–25.

Liebenhagen, A. and Forsberg, A. (2013) 'The courage to surrender – placing one's life in the hands of the other', *Journal of Perianesthesia Nursing*, 28(5): 271–282.

Link, B. and Streuning, E. (1997) 'On stigma and its consequences: Evidence from a longitudinal study of men with dual diagnosis of mental and substance abuse', *Journal of Health and Social Behaviour*, 38: 177–190.

Lopez, S.J., O'Byrne, K.K. and Petersen, S. (2003) 'Profiling courage', in S.J. Lopez and C.R. Snyder (eds), *Positive Psychological Assessment: A Handbook of Models and Measures*. Washington, DC: American Psychological Association. pp. 185–197.

Magnano, P., Paolillo, A., Platania, S. and Santisi, G. (2017) 'Courage as a potential mediator between personality and coping', *Personality and Individual Differences*, 111: 13–18.

Mandell, A.M. and Green, R.C. (2011) 'Alzheimer's disease', in A.E. Budson and N.W. Kowall (eds), *The Handbook of Alzheimer's Disease and Other Dementias*. In D. Mostofsky (series ed.), *Handbooks of Behavioural Neuroscience*. Chichester, UK: Wiley-Blackwell. pp. 3–92.

May, R. (1977) *The Meaning of Anxiety*. London: Norton & Co.

McCartney, M. (2014) 'Courage is treating patients with Ebola', *BMJ*, 349: g4987.

McDowell, S.E. and Ferner, R.E. (2013) 'Medical manslaughter', *BMJ*, 347: f5609.

McKeon, R.P.E. (1941) *The Basic Works of Aristotle*. New York: Random House.

Meissner, H.I., et al. (1992) 'How sources of health information relate to knowledge about use of cancer-screening exams', *Journal of Community Health*, 17: 153–165.

Meyer, E.C. (2014) 'Courage, brains and heart: Lessons from the Wizard of Oz for difficult healthcare conversations', *Australian Critical Care*, 27(3): 108–109.

Moules, N.J., Simonson, K., Fleiszer, A.R., Prins, M. and Glasgow, Rev B. (2007) 'The soul of sorrow work: Grief and therapeutic interventions with families', *Journal of Family Nursing*, 13(1): 117–141.

Mu, P.F., Lee, M.Y., Sheng, C.C., Tung, P.C., Huang, L.Y. and Chen, Y.W. (2015) 'The experiences of family members in the year following the diagnosis of a child or adolescent with cancer: A qualitative systematic review', *JBI Database of Systematic Reviews and Implementation Reports*, 13(5): 293–329.

Naef, R. (2006) 'Bearing witness: A moral way of engaging in the nurse–person relationship', *Nursing Philosophy*, 7(3): 146–156.

National Institute for Health and Care Excellence (NICE) (2014) *Safe Staffing for Nursing in Adult Inpatient Wards in Acute Hospitals*. Safe staffing guideline No 1. London: NICE.

Norton, P.J. and Weiss, B.J. (2009) 'The role of courage on behavioral approach in a fear-eliciting situation: A proof-of-concept pilot study', *Journal of Anxiety Disorders*, 23(2): 212–217.

Peters-Golden, H. (1982) 'Breast cancer: Varied perceptions of social support in the illness experience', *Social Science & Medicine*, 16: 483–491.

Quick, O. (2017) 'Medical manslaughter – time for a rethink?', *Medico-Legal Journal*, 85(4): 173–181.

Reason, J.T. (2000) 'Human error: Models and management', *BMJ*, 320.

Recio-Saucedo, A., Pope, C., Dall'Ora, C., Griffiths, P., Jones, J., Crouch, R. and Drennan, J. (2015) 'Safe staffing for nursing in emergency departments: Evidence review', *Emergency Medicine Journal*, 32(11): 888–894.

Rock, L. (2018) 'Interview: When do you know you're old enough to die? Barbara Ehrenreich has some answers', *The Guardian*, 7 April. Available at: www.theguardian.com/lifeandstyle/2018/apr/07/barbara-ehrenreich-natural-causes-book-old-enough-to-die (accessed 5 June 2018).

Rohde, G., Kersten, C., Vistad, I. and Mesel, T. (2017) 'Spiritual well-being in patients with metastatic colorectal cancer receiving noncurative chemotherapy: A qualitative study', *Cancer Nursing, 40*(3): 209–216.

Rushton, C., Halifax, J. and Dossey, B. (2007) 'Being with dying, contemplative practices for compassionate end of-life care', *American Nurse Today, 2*(9): 16–18.

Rydé, K., Strang, P. and Friedrichsen, M. (2008) 'Crying in solitude or with someone for support and consolation – experiences from family members in palliative home care', *Cancer Nursing, 31*(5): 345–353.

Sacks, O. (2015) *My Own Life: Oliver Sacks on Learning he has Terminal Cancer.* Available at: www.nytimes.com/2015/02/19/opinion/oliver-sacks-on-learning-he-has-terminal-cancer.html (accessed 5 June 2018).

Savickas, M.L. (2015) 'Life design with adults: Developmental individualization using biographical bricolage', in L. Nota and J. Rossier (eds), *Handbook of Life Design: From Practice to Theory and from Theory to Practice.* Göttingen: Hogrefe. pp. 135–150.

Seale, C. (2002) 'Cancer heroics: A study of news reports with particular reference to gender', *Sociology, 36*(1): 107–126.

Smith, R. (2000) 'A good death', *BMJ, 320*(7228): 129–130.

Swaffer, K. (2016) *What the Hell Happened to my Brain?* London: Jessica-Kingsley Publishers.

Tee, N. (2003) *Resilience and Courage: Women, Men and the Holocaust.* New Haven, CT: Yale University Press.

Tillich, P. (1952) *The Courage to Be.* New Haven, NY: Yale University Press.

Titcombe, J. (2015) *Joshua's Story.* Leeds: Anderson Wallace Publishing.

Titcombe, J. (2017) 'It's too late for my son, but the end of the campaign for "normal birth" is welcome', *The Guardian*, 14 August. Available at: www.theguardian.com/commentis-free/2017/aug/14/royal-college-midwives-normal-birth-joshua-titcombe (accessed 5 June 2018).

Tornøe, K.A., Danbolt, L.J., Kvigne, K. and Sørlie, V. (2014) 'The power of consoling presence – hospice nurses' lived experience with spiritual and existential care for the dying', *BMC Nursing, 13*: 25 doi: 10.1186/1472–6955–13–25.

Tsai, T.J., Chung, U.L., Chang, C.J. and Wang, H.H. (2016) 'Influence of religious beliefs on the health of cancer patients', *Asian Pacific Journal of Cancer Prevention, 17*(4): 2315–2320.

Van Gorp, B. and Vercruysse, T. (2012) 'Frames and counter-frames giving meaning to dementia: A framing analysis of media content', *Social Science & Medicine, 74*: 1274–1281.

Webster, G. and Bayliss, F. (2000) 'Moral residue', in S.B. Rubin and L. Zoloth (eds), *Margin of Error: The Ethics of Mistakes in the Practice of Medicine.* Hagerstown, MD: University Publishing Group.

Wilkinson, J.P. (2016) 'Courage', *BJOG, 123*(8): 1393.

Woodard, C. (2004) 'Hardiness and the concept of courage', *Consulting Psychology Journal: Practice and Research, 56*(3): 173–185.

Woodgate, R.L. and Busolo, D.S. (2017) 'Healthy Canadian adolescents' perspectives of cancer using metaphors: A qualitative study', *BMJ Open, 7*(1): e013958.

Wright, L. M. (2005) *Spirituality, Suffering and Illness: Ideas for Healing.* Philadelphia: E A Davis.

Zeilig, H. (2014) 'Dementia as a cultural metaphor', *Gerontologist, 54*(2): 258–267.

5

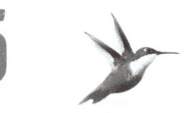

COURAGE TO CHALLENGE

SHIBLEY RAHMAN

Introduction

Feedback has been implicated in the theory of control systems for a very long time. Behaviours occasionally need to be challenged for systems to learn. A 'courage to challenge' has been framed by the CIPD as a situation where someone 'shows courage and confidence to speak up skilfully, challenging others even when confronted with resistance or unfamiliar circumstances' (see www.cipd.co.uk/Images/Courage-to-Challenge_tcm18-9692.pdf). Such a person making a challenge 'takes a stand and acts on their own beliefs, despite significant opposition and personal risk' and 'stands up for self and the organisation publicly when the worst happens in difficult circumstances …'.

But if the environment demands a strong and robust challenge, in the face of an environment hostile to criticism and/or where criticism is not perceived as needed, 'whistleblowing' may be required. We indeed have a lot to be grateful to 'whistleblowers' for, generally, both within the NHS and social care and far beyond. For example, only very recently, Christopher Wylie 'became famous' as a Canadian whistleblower in the Facebook and Cambridge Analytica data breach. The documents allegedly centre around Cambridge Analytica's alleged unauthorised possession of personal private data from some 50 million Facebook user accounts, obtained for the purpose of creating targeted political campaigns for the 2016 US presidential elections. Wylie writes himself:

> I'm disappointed, but I also understand it. It is extremely uncomfortable to consider that our democracy may have been corrupted. That potential crimes may have taken place – some of them on Facebook's servers – that seem to be beyond the reach of law. It's why I testified last week to parliament. It's why I have given three binders of evidence about Vote Leave to the UK Electoral Commission and information commissioner's office. (Wylie, 2018)

We know that within health and social care challenging can be difficult, especially if there are rigid, formal hierarchies at play; however, a lack of ability to challenge runs the risk of worsening performance of services as a whole.

The close link between bullying and sickness rates within the NHS is truly alarming. According to a report by NHS Employers, on average 71% of people who were bullied felt worried about going to work, while nearly a fifth took time off as a direct result. There, arguably, needs to be a frank admission that sickness might be linked to the culture of an organisation (Jolliff, 2016). This brings into play two further issues of whether the workforce budgets are adequate, and whether unwell staff can look after unwell patients. How much courage is needed by individual members of the workforce to 'keep going' is a worrying issue, which many people do not wish to discuss openly.

This chapter will focus on the issues faced by whistleblowers, although it has to be noted that this forms only one manifestation of a 'courage to challenge' in the NHS and social care. Whistleblowers have a critical role in setting the moral compass of the NHS and social care, and courage is critical to this.

Giacalone and Promislo (2013) argue that, whether implicitly or explicitly, much scholarship in business ethics has assumed that all individuals wish to (or can be convinced to) engage in and support ethical decisions and decision makers but, unfortunately, this assumption needs rigorous scrutiny. Research shows us that ethical behaviour, whether framed within philosophy or other domains, such as positive psychology (Snyder and Lopez, 2002), is often undermined and is not necessarily a priority for some persons and organisations. All organisations have 'grey areas' where the border between 'right' and 'wrong' behaviour is blurred, but where a major part of organisational decision making takes place. While grey areas can be sources of problems for organisations, they also potentially have benefits or present opportunities. Grey areas can become problematic when the process for dealing with them is flawed, for example when leaders, perhaps by their own inattention, inaction and poor modelling, minimise the importance of building a moral community by delegating grey area issues to 'middle managers' (Bruhn, 2009).

One often wonders whether hard-working staff in any organisation actually set out to be 'evil' or 'malicious'. It is said that the risk of corruption is significantly heightened in environments where the reporting of wrongdoing is not supported or protected. Both public and private sector employees have access to up-to-date information concerning their workplaces' practices, and are usually the first to recognise wrongdoings. 'Speak-up' arrangements can have economic benefits for organisations and society.

So what exactly is whistleblowing?

'Whistleblowing' itself sounds like a harsh and pejorative term, but is important from a societal and an ethical perspective; it also saves money both for private and public sector organisations. A recent study of over 5000 firms showed that 40% of companies surveyed suffered from serious economic crimes that averaged over $3m each in losses (Devine, 2012). Whistleblowing is the term used 'when someone who works for an employer raises a concern about malpractice, risk (for example about patient safety), wrongdoing or possible illegality, which harms, or creates a risk of harm, to people who use the service, colleagues or the wider public' (Care Quality Commission, 2013: 3).

Definitions of 'whistleblowing' vary across sectors and jurisdictions. Firtko and Jackson, for example, have defined whistleblowing as: 'the reporting of information to an individual, group, or body that is not part of an organisation's usual problem solving strategy ... a phenomenon where a party or parties take matters that would normally be held as confidential to an organisation outside the organisation despite the personal risk and potentially negative sequales associated with the act' (2005: 52).

Whistleblowing can occur outside the NHS and social care, and is still instructive here arguably. Whistleblowing, which takes enormous courage, most agree, can be pivotal in stopping misfeasance and misconduct. For example, in many African countries, 'the secretive and self-serving deeds of political and business elites have come to light thanks only to whistleblowers' (Garzón and Bourdon, 2017). In yet another recent whistleblower case, Daniel Donovan, an information manager at Volkswagen, filed a lawsuit claiming he was unlawfully fired because people at the company feared that he was going to report to authorities the destruction of documents related to VW's installation of illegal software on diesel engines in order to cheat on emissions tests (he later withdrew the case after what some suspect was a private settlement) (Ewing, 2016).

NHS England (2016) in Clauses 1.1.3 to 1.1.15 of *Voicing Your Concerns for Staff (Whistleblowing Policy)* describe their commitment to protecting whistleblowers who raise 'relevant concerns' in the 'public interest', in keeping with the NHS constitution and NHS values. The NHS Constitution for England (Department of Health, 2015) sets out the principles, values and rights of patients and staff with regard to raising concerns in the NHS. It makes a number of pledges, the most notable of which can be found in Section 4b, 'Staff – your responsibilities'. It is stated that staff should aim 'to provide all patients with safe care, and to do all you can to protect patients from harm' (2015: 14). It has, however, long been recognised that whistleblowing and how it influences the individual, their family, work colleagues, nursing practice and policy overall, requires further national and international research attention (Jackson et al., 2014).

Examples of well-known NHS and social care whistleblowers

Whistleblowers in the health and social care world, especially in the NHS, undoubtedly need to have huge courage. This involves doing something perceived for the greater good, while often jeopardising and threatening their own personal and professional existence in an act of apparent self-destruction. Examples of whistleblowers in the NHS and social care appear to have common strands. The outcomes for whistleblowers, despite their enormous courage, are, on the whole, depressingly bad. Case studies 5.1 to 5.6 are brief accounts of 'real' whistleblowers, and the descriptions are based on publicly available published accounts.

Case study 5.1: Dr Raj Mattu

An NHS whistleblower, a cardiologist called Dr Raj Mattu, who was unfairly sacked after exposing concerns about patient safety, was awarded £1.22m in damages by a hospital trust. Mattu claimed he had been vilified and bullied, and subjected to a 12-year 'witch-hunt' after making the claims in 2001. He was sacked in 2010, but a Birmingham employment tribunal ruled that he had been unfairly dismissed (Press Association, 2016).

In April 2001 Dr Raj Mattu and five colleagues sounded the alarm about what they said was the dangerous 'five in four' practice at Walsgrave Hospital in Coventry of putting a fifth bed in a bay of a cardiac ward only designed to take four. Their concerns – that the practice would leave vital services such as oxygen, suction and mains electricity harder to reach in the event of an emergency – appeared, it is alleged, to be borne out when a patient suffered a heart attack and died after staff could not reach that equipment in time. Mattu exposed the cases of two patients who had died in crowded bays at Walsgrave Hospital in Coventry (*BBC News*, 2016).

Those concerns led to a chain of events which ended with Mattu's sacking by University Hospitals Coventry and Warwickshire NHS Trust in 2010, but an employment tribunal in April ruled that Mattu had been unfairly dismissed. His former NHS trust is reported to have spent £6m pursuing about 200 allegations against him.

Case study 5.2: Dr Chris Day

A junior doctor 'blew the whistle' about unsafe staffing levels at his hospital and won a potential landmark legal victory in the fight for better protections for medics who raise concerns in the workplace. Dr Chris Day had discovered that 54,000 NHS doctors in training appear not to have any 'whistleblowing protection' if they dared to speak up and are punished as a result. He claims his career was destroyed after he raised concerns over staffing levels on the Intensive Care Unit at Queen Elizabeth Hospital in Woolwich, south-east London, where he worked in 2014. He reported he had been forced to cover extra wards, including A&E, after two locum doctors failed to turn up. Lewisham and Greenwich NHS Trust has accepted that a protected disclosure about

(Continued)

(Continued)

safety and staffing was made to it on the night of 10 January 2014, but his contract was terminated and his career path to consultant was stalled.

In May 2016, his case against Health Education England, which arranges junior doctors' training contracts, was thrown out by the Employment Appeal Tribunal. It ruled that he could not claim whistleblower protection against HEE because the trust with which he was placed, not HEE, was his employer. Three senior judges then at the Court of Appeal held that the appeal tribunal was wrong to decide that the trust was his sole employer (Dyer, 2017). The judges ruled that the HEE – which arranges junior doctors' training contracts, pays a substantial part of their salaries and reviews their progress in training – could also be considered an employer. In an agency arrangement, both the 'introducer' and the 'end user' could be an employer under the wording of the Employment Rights Act 1996, the judges said. Day has had issues finding subsequent employment in the NHS.

Case study 5.3: Dr Stephen Bolsin

Stephen Bolsin, 63, is another prime example of the NHS whistleblowing experience, as the man who blew the whistle on failings in paediatric heart surgery at Bristol Royal Infirmary and was rewarded with the sound of slamming doors (*BMJ*, 2016). As an anaesthetist appointed as a consultant in Bristol in 1988, Bolsin recognised and tried to remedy failings in the service, finally turning 'whistleblower'. This led to the Kennedy inquiry, which vindicated his concerns and was a landmark in clinical governance. He subsequently found it impossible to find another position in the UK and moved to Australia, where he became director of critical care services at Geelong Hospital in Victoria, achieving world-class outcomes with the adult cardiac anaesthetic service he started.

Case study 5.4: Dr Kim Holt

A consultant paediatrician who raised concerns about a clinic where baby Peter Connelly was treated days before his death has warned that the NHS still has a culture where managers and organisations are stopping potential whistleblowers from speaking out (Mooney, 2011). Dr Kim Holt, who raised concerns over poor record keeping and understaffing at St Ann's Clinic in Haringey, north London, where Peter Connelly was seen by an inexperienced locum doctor at the clinic days before he was killed, told the *BMJ* that whistleblowers were often being 'gagged' by clauses written into their contracts after they are 'paid off by NHS organisations to leave their jobs'.

The case of 'Baby P' has profound repercussions about the culture of working in health and social care, both of which can be dominated by toxic hierarchies.

> Learning from the case of 'Baby P' is vitally important. Knowledge of how the complexities of the politics of blame, fear and denial functioned in the case is instructive. Blame, fear and denial need now to be replaced by knowledge, awareness and understanding to achieve a renewed focus on how cases of familial child homicide are managed. I believe that it is only the social work profession itself that can transcend the blame, fear and denial that characterised the responses to the familial homicide of Peter Connelly. (Shoesmith, 2016: 224)

Case study 5.5:   Dr David Drew

A former clinical director of Walsall Manor Hospital, Dr David Drew was dismissed in December 2010 after voicing concerns about what he said was a huge cost-cutting exercise. The consultant paediatrician, a Christian, fell foul of his trust after including a biblical reference in an email to several fellow doctors as part of an attempt to lift their spirits.

He was ultimately sacked for 'gross misconduct and insubordination' after he refused to accept the findings of a review panel that investigated his behaviour. The email was a smokescreen to justify getting rid of him, Drew said. Drew lost an employment tribunal appeal of unfair dismissal in 2013, but maintains that he was sacked for his whistleblowing activities.

Drew writes, 'Sharing the stories of others was sobering. So many had worse experiences than me. They were all first-class health professionals, honest to the core and excellent communicators' (2014: 292).

Case study 5.6:   Sharmila Chowdhury

Finally, a radiographer Sharmila Chowdhury was suspended by Ealing Hospital in West London after raising concerns in 2007 that colleagues were moonlighting at a nearby private hospital, a practice that was costing the NHS trust a huge amount of money. Despite winning her case at an interim relief tribunal in 2010, the trust refused to take her back. Chowdhury has not worked in the NHS since then, despite having worked in the service for 27 years before her suspension. She has spent more than £130,000 in legal fees pursuing her case. 'Despite winning a hearing in which I was proven to be a whistleblower, I've no job and no money', she is reported to have said.

Whistleblowing and the courage needed for it is an incredibly interesting subject cognitively, emotionally and behaviourally. Needham (2012) sees little virtue in the term 'whistleblowing' itself, where 'problems remain with the negative connotations of the term "whistleblowing"'. Perhaps it might indeed be time for a new word? Organisational ethics scholars have recognised the need to encourage the development of moral strength in the workplace and that this will require more than a superficial re-invention of programmes, policies and penalties (Verschoor, 2004). Whistleblowing, then, is often fraught with rival interpretations and always happens in a deeply cultural and highly situated organisational context. In analysing and implanting a strategy for enabling people to challenge safely (and, at one extreme, to 'blow the whistle'), it is therefore difficult to make cross-jurisdictional comparisons, because of differences in, for example, political, social and legal infrastructures. Organisational policies thus need very careful design, implementation and enacting to protect those raising legitimate concerns as well as offering support in cases of fallout from more vexatious whistleblowing.

All of the real examples above are of people who sat in the 'middle' of the organisation but speaking out can happen at the top of organisations too, as the fictional example of Stephanie below shows.

Example from Practice 5.1

Stephanie, Director of Nursing, University Teaching Hospital

Stephanie was a Director of Nursing in a large University Teaching Hospital and the executive lead for quality and safety. Part of her role was to review the morbidity and mortality data and to ensure that any abnormalities in trends were fully investigated, lessons learnt and changes made.

During her time in this post it became clear that there was a worrying trend of increased morbidity within one of the specialities and a number of unexpected deaths. Further investigation identified these outcomes were patients under the care of two consultants.

In discussion with the medical director it was agreed to do an in-depth review of all aspects of the care to understand what was happening and the root cause.

In response to the request for further data from the speciality team the Director of Nursing (DON) started to get several uncomfortable emails and comments about her role in looking at this and felt that she was being asked to leave this to local management which she felt uncomfortable about.

Concern began to surface about the level of experience and qualifications of the doctors in question which she repeatedly raised, and again she experienced some push back about her suitability to make that judgement.

Pressure started to be placed on the DON that her persistence on this issue was causing difficulties within the organisation and 'making her difficult to work with'.

She was advised that it would be 'helpful' if she started to think about her next career move, with a conversation with the CEO that a move to another provider organisation might be sensible.

During this time the DON was checking her data and concerns with other medical colleagues and the commissioner to establish whether she was misinterpreting data and to act as a sounding board. Her concerns and interpretations were verified by external sources, which gave her the strength to continue to push the agenda.

After several months of pushing, the situation became untenable and she was told she would be dismissed if she did not leave. She agreed to leave subject to a compromise agreement, which explicitly included an external review of the service and outcomes. This was agreed and both the medics in question were subsequently suspended from the organisation and dismissed.

Reflections on Stephanie's experience: When exploring what enabled Stephanie to pursue the issue, she described an unwavering push to protect patients in the face of evidence to the contrary, a signed commitment that action would be taken, psychological, social and economic resources to provide an infrastructure for her and a strong value base to 'do the right thing'.

General problems faced by whistleblowers

Healthcare scandals in many countries have demonstrated that uncaring and ineffective practices can flourish if the organisational context goes wrong (Braithwaite et al., 2015). Managers tasked with clinical governance must be aware of mechanisms which conspire to minimise the effect of dealing with 'negative feedback'. The human tendency to favour positive news and avoid conflict is powerful.

We first introduced wilful blindness in Chapter 3. Understanding wilful blindness can assist managers' awareness of the competing emotions occurring in response to ethical challenges, such as whistleblowing (Cleary and Duke, 2017). Research suggests that those who know most about wrongdoing are often those closest to the action (Armstrong and Francis, 2014). These people have been termed 'whistleblowers' if they decide to report the wrongdoing.

'Blowing the whistle', however, is fraught with risks and this is increasingly recognised by the widespread adoption of whistleblower legislation to protect the whistleblower. Across various jurisdictions, the law has to allow a delicate balance between protecting the whistleblower with genuine measures and not opening the floodgates for vexatious complaints which would become unmanageable for the employer. Even in the US, although whistleblowing has been deeply culturally ingrained since the Lloyd-La Follette Act (1912), individuals remain vulnerable to bullying and gagging. The Act was created by Congress in response to the issuance of executive orders by

Presidents Theodore Roosevelt and William H. Taft that forbade federal employees from communicating directly with Congress without the permission of their supervisors. In a recent case uncovered by medical journals, two Texas nurses were criminally prosecuted for reporting a doctor to the state medical board over patient safety (Braillon and Bewley, 2015).

'The whistleblower speaks out about illegal or unethical behaviour within his or her organisation' (Alford, 1999: 266). Such 'speaking out' is often discussed in the context of (business) ethics where it appears as a 'moral duty' (Vandekerckhove and Tsahuridu, 2010); as an expression of 'ethical autonomy' (Alford, 2001). In England, the 'Francis Report' identified staff who were scared to speak out, and when they did, senior staff were hostile towards them and defensive of existing practices. This fits with the old adage that staff should 'give in or get out': giving in and accepting the status quo is easier than getting out (Hilton, 2016). The report states, 'Many described a harrowing and isolating process with reprisals including counter allegations, disciplinary action, and victimisation. Bullying and oppressive behaviour was mentioned frequently, both as a subject for concern and a consequence of speaking up' (cited in https://thepsychologist.bps.org.uk/whistleblowers-heroes-not-headaches). The report said that accounts from people who related their experiences to the review contained more references to bullying than to any other problem. Francis recommended that failure to modify bullying behaviour should always be a matter for disciplinary action (Dyer, 2015).

As well as facing disciplinary action, whistleblowers may find themselves referred by employers to their professional regulator. Francis said that regulators such as the General Medical Council need to ascertain any risk that a referral may be 'retaliatory'. In NHS organisations, responsibility for whistleblowing should be removed from human resources departments and made part of incident reporting, arguably. The frequency of victimisation against whistleblowers has reportedly ranged from a high of about 90% down to 22% (Bowden, 2014). Bowden notes that victimisation may be reducing over time as the higher rates are from older studies. As policies and legislation are now in place to protect whistleblowers from such behaviour and the use of internal whistleblowing systems has developed, whistleblowing may be perceived as an important element in improving organisational governance. The obligations of employees are typically held to include a duty to avoid doing things that would harm the employer's interests, for example by damaging the employer's reputation, or by exposing proprietary information that might give an advantage to competitors. Employers are (understandably) only able to entrust sensitive information to employees on the condition that they will keep this information confidential (MacDougall, 2016).

Although the notion of safety culture remains problematic in terms of definition and implementation, 'the way things are done around here' – probably the simplest explanation of what safety culture means (Reason, 1998) – has changed and there is a considered and sustained drive to enhance the quality and safety of healthcare provision. Concrete evidence of organisational environments in healthcare, which prospectively learn from staff concerns, can be seen outside of the United Kingdom. For example, the Patient Safety Alert (PSA) system designed by Virginia Mason Medical

Center in Seattle, WA, USA has transformed the working environment. Although the PSA system initially focused only on actual lapses or near misses in safety and medical error, a PSA is now intended to capture all events involving the safety and wellbeing of a patient such as medication errors and grade 3 to 4 pressure ulcers, elevators not working properly and disruptive behaviours of staff and patient (Jones, 2015).

The 'sound of silence'

In law, across various jurisdictions, it is not entirely consistent when silence can be deemed to constitute acceptance. The social virtues of silence are reinforced by instincts for survival and self-preservation, arguably. Many organisations send out the message – verbally or non-verbally – that falling into line is the safest way to hold on to our jobs and further our careers. The need for quiet submission is exaggerated by today's difficult economy, where millions of people have lost their jobs and many more worry that they might (Perlow and Williams, 2003). Whilst not all incidents result in patient harm, there is increasing recognition that 'open disclosure' about any incident that occurs or may occur is intrinsic to good quality care, and is becoming an expected aspect of patient involvement (Iedema et al., 2009). Numerous definitions of whistleblowing appear in healthcare and business literature, but all point to the importance of advocacy, that is, protecting someone who will likely be harmed. For this book, the definition will differentiate between reporting the problem within the organisation and whistleblowing to an external agency (Fletcher et al., 1998; Sellin, 1995). It has been mooted that advocacy in nursing has its origins in the teachings of Florence Nightingale which are inherently moral and good (Watson and O'Connor, 2017).

Studies have suggested that some organisations might have violated basic ethical standards and betrayed our trust. Huberts (2014) noted that almost half of US workers reported seeing one or more acts of wrongdoing (e.g. accepting 'kickbacks' or bribes, offering bribes to public officials, lying to outside stakeholders, environmental violations) on the job within the past year. Research for the Institute of Business Ethics has shown that while one in four employees is aware of misconduct at work, more than half (52%) of those stay silent. Organisations that can overcome this culture of silence by encouraging openness are likely to benefit in a number of ways.

It is argued that an organisation where the value of 'open whistleblowing' is recognised will be better able to:

- deter wrongdoing
- pick up problems early
- enable critical information to get to the people who need to know and can address the issue
- demonstrate to stakeholders, regulators and the courts that they are accountable and well managed
- reduce the risk of anonymous and malicious leaks

- minimise costs and compensation from accidents, investigations, litigation and regulatory inspections
- maintain and enhance its reputation.

Most often 'silence' comes across as the option of least risk for the employee, as well as the employer, who encounters fraud or corruption. It is an attractive option for various reasons. Most often the whistleblower fears harsh criticism, or feels that there could be a simple explanation to it. The individual may also question why he/she should point it out when others who are also aware, are not raising concerns. On the other hand, in organisations where fraud and corruption are common practice, the whistleblower himself might be expected to prove his point rather than witnessing justice through an investigation. This again would discourage a whistleblower. For example, in the Clapham rail crash of 1988, the Inquiry into the crash found that workers knew that there was risky loose wiring but had turned a blind eye. In the gas leak of Union Carbide India in 1984, workers, together with a local journalist, had raised concerns, but these had been ignored by the local authority.

Clinical governance and the regulators

Research by healthcare professionals and specifically nurses has shown that whistle-blowing is considered to have occurred only when referring to external disclosures. Additionally prior to reporting externally, the *would-be* whistleblower should have exhausted all the internal reporting mechanisms in order to effect action to bring to an end the offending practice. The clear distinction in health service literature that whistleblowing only includes external disclosures arises from the need to value internal reporting of error and misconduct as a 'normal' organisational process (clinical governance), which does not involve a breach of confidentiality commonly associated with reporting to an unauthorised external authority (Cleary and Doyle, 2016). Yet numerous surveys across different professional groups highlight a disconnect between whistleblowing policies in theory and how such arrangements work in practice.

One possible reason for this is the widely held perception among health professionals that they will be victimised, ostracised or bullied if they raise legitimate concerns about the work of colleagues or about poor care. The General Medical Council (GMC) and other regulators recognise the importance of speaking up to protect patient safety. All health professionals have a duty to do so. The fact that it remains risky and difficult is little short of scandalous. There has been consistently reported a culture of bullying when doctors try to speak up, and Holt confirms that: 'An employer might use the process of making an allegation to the GMC about a doctor's fitness to practise as an act of retaliation against a doctor because he or she raised concerns, or, simply, as an inappropriate alternative to dealing with the matter in-house' (Holt, 2015).

The GMC's core guidance in *Good Medical Practice* provides a number of critical clauses which specify what registered doctors must do in certain conditions, such as if there are insufficient resources in a place of work, or if a colleague might be deemed unfit to practise (for example, due to ill health). The exact wording of the code of conduct should be read carefully (GMC, 2014).

In his famous reports, Sir Robert Francis QC had noted particular challenges in primary care because many staff work in small teams, which makes it harder to raise concerns confidentially or anonymously. Primary care staff may also be worried about raising concerns about someone who is a direct employer. The primary care workforce includes certain groups who are particularly vulnerable, such as temporary staff, locums and students, as they may be in practices only for short periods of time (Wise, 2016). Ethical breakdowns in corporate America not only hurt the US economy but also harm the integrity of businesses in the eyes of their many stakeholders. Unfortunately, there are many recent examples of such malfeasance: Enron and the International Olympic Committee are just two famous examples (Calvert, 2002). Together, these studies suggest that rebels are resented when their implicit reproach threatens the positive self-image of those individuals who did not rebel.

Despite reported concerns about the quality of care and the existence of professional codes and organisational guidelines in many organisations, under-reporting of problems/concerns (for example, incompetent, unethical or illegal behaviour) are the norm (Firth-Cozens et al., 2003). The study of Firth-Cozens and colleagues with nurses working in the NHS indicated that only 63% of those who observed poor care reported it. Literature on patient safety confirms this tendency to under-report poor care (Runciman et al., 1998; Vincent et al., 1999; Meurier, 2000; Wakefield and Maddox, 2000). There is a dilemma for nurses when misconduct occurs. In this situation nurses are faced with two options: they can report the misconduct or remain silent. Responses to an anonymous survey of nurses indicated that 'both options cause physical and emotional effects' (McDonald and Ahern, 2000: 313–321). The survey from Firth-Cozens and colleagues, completed in the NHS in 2003, showed that 29 out of the 35 subjects who had blown the whistle in their organisations had an average of 5.3 symptoms at the time of the survey, the most common symptoms being sleep problems, panic attacks, depression and feelings of guilt and unworthiness. Moore and McAuliffe (2010) conducted a study of 152 nurses in Irish hospitals and highlighted the culture of silence in hospitals and the poor organisational response to whistleblowers as critical issues that need to be addressed in order to encourage whistleblowing.

When to 'blow the whistle', moral distress and moral courage

Many strong predictors of whether a worker will decide to blow the whistle or not are determined by the worker's organisation, including organisational support and encouragement for whistleblowing, dissemination of knowledge about the proper avenues for reporting unethical behaviour, and clear safety measures to protect whistleblowers from retaliation (Dungan et al., 2015). In addition, situational factors that increase the salience of the act's severity facilitate 'blowing the whistle' – people are more likely to voice disapproval of others' behaviour when that behaviour becomes unethical abruptly rather than slowly over time (Gino and Bazerman, 2009). Effective voicing of concerns is but the first stage in reshaping better, safer healthcare; those with influence have to hear, and they have to act. In the management literature, the concept of the 'deaf effect' has been defined as occurring when 'the decision-maker does not hear, ignores or overrules a report of bad news to continue a failing course of action' (Cueller et al., 2006). Mansbach and colleagues (2012) added that the likelihood of junior staff and learners speaking out, is entirely dependent on whether the voice and actions of all staff (irrespective of grade) are actively encouraged and valued by the organisation.

Demonstrating whistleblowers are not 'intrinsically different' from non-whistleblowers is part of the removal of justification for ignoring reports of wrongdoing (Cassematis and Wortley, 2013). There is a reason to believe that whistleblowers are not markedly different from non-reporting colleagues. For example, Somers and Casal (1994) found whistleblowers had neither particularly high nor particularly low organisational commitment. Although the general perception is that courage has costs, research led by David Mayer (2016) suggests that that conclusion should be more nuanced. People tend to denigrate their peers for speaking up because it is not viewed as their place, but they celebrate leaders who do so because they expect them to be the moral voice of organisations. An important implication of this research is that leaders have a critical responsibility both to speak up and to create a culture where employees are accountable to one another and the organisation to report any wrongdoing. Of critical importance is how in any organisational culture the ethical leadership is communicated to employees to promote values effectively, to encourage compliance (Killingsworth, 2012). It seems that employees not only judge the ethical legitimacy of authority from formal communications received in the workplace but also from actual behaviour and conduct.

Moral courage is the ability to rise above fear and take action based on one's ethical beliefs (Lachman, 2007). Discussions among diverse groups of rural and urban healthcare professionals and patients can foster a unified understanding of the politics, emotions and values that continue to impair moral courage and ethical action (Aultman, 2008). For example, in deciding whether to 'whistleblow', the nurse could ask, 'Am I comfortable with this decision?' As Gen. Morrison said in a 2013 address:

> The standard you walk past is the standard you accept. That goes for all of us, but especially those who by their rank have a leadership role. If we are a great national institution, if we care about the legacy left to us by those who served before us, if we care about the legacy we leave to those who, in turn, will protect and secure Australia, then it is up to us to make a difference. If you're not up to it, find something else to do with your life. There is no place for you amongst this band of brothers and sisters.

MacDonald (2002) offered some help with this. The nurse may not be 'comfortable' because often situations requiring the virtue of integrity and courage are not comfortable at the time. However, it is imperative that the nurse ask questions like the following to determine if, in the long term, he or she could continue in the profession while maintaining a high level of integrity:

1. If I carry out this decision, would I be comfortable telling my family about it?
2. Would I want my children to take my behaviour as an example?
3. Is this decision one which a wise, informed, virtuous person would make?
4. Can I live with my decision?

Moral distress has been discussed in the field of healthcare (Kalvemark et al., 2004), but it is also relevant to social work practice. Moral distress begins when a social worker's personal and professional values collide with agency policies or expectations. Ethical dilemmas, when left unresolved, ultimately create moral distress: 'A situation that might present a dilemma for one person (a difficult choice between two equally unwelcome courses of action), might for another be an ethical problem (the situation is difficult, but it is clear what choice should be made), or might even be regarded as devoid of ethical content' (Banks, 2001). Not everyone cares about doing the right thing, possibly due to an inherent 'standard' of morality. The practice of courage is an important trait for members of any organisation (Verschoor, 2003), and an important quality or attribute necessary for ethical behaviour in organisational settings (Hesselbein, 2005; Pears, 2004). Courage has been described as a management virtue (Srivastva and Cooperrider, 1998), with professional courage depicted as an attribute that motivates and enables individuals to take the right course of action, given the ethics of their profession (Harris, 1999).

'Moral courage' bridges the gap between knowing one's personal values and professional obligations, and acting on them despite risks such as social ostracism, embarrassment or loss of employment (Aultman, 2008; Lachman, 2007). For morally courageous individuals, upholding their core values is judged worth exposing themselves to harm or vulnerability (Lachman, 2010). The majority of students who are faced with moral dilemmas, choose to remain silent for a myriad of reasons (Bradbury-Jones et al., 2007; Rees et al., 2015). Whilst some students may subsequently report the behaviour (Rees et al., 2015), at the time of the event, they often remain passive spectators and sometimes even active participants (Grealish and Trevitt, 2005; Levett-Jones and Lathlean, 2009). Fear of punitive action and disproportionate apportionment of blame also continue to inhibit nurse involvement (Luk et al., 2008; Shannon et al., 2009).

Since 2014, the NHS has had to comply with a statutory 'duty of candour'. We first introduced this as a professional concept in Chapter 1. This means that staff must be honest with patients and their families when an untoward incident, for which they are responsible, causes physical or 'prolonged psychological' harm or death (Hilton, 2016). The government has placed a new legal duty on all organisations to ensure that, when something goes wrong, patients and their relatives are told about it promptly. Known as the Duty of Candour, it is intended to counteract the legalistic and defensive culture that was found at Mid Staffordshire, fostering instead a culture in which mistakes are acknowledged and learned from. The professional regulators, such as the General Medical Council and the Nursing and Midwifery Council, are introducing consistent responsibilities on individual health professionals so that action can be taken when they are not candid about errors with their patients. This professional accountability is being reinforced through the introduction of the role of the 'responsible clinician' (Department of Health, 2015).

The current legal framework

Certainly English law is in a state of flux over whistleblowing. The Public Interest Disclosure Act 1998 (PIDA), which introduced the 'whistleblowing' provisions in the Employment Rights Act 1996, was enacted against the backdrop of a series of scandals and disasters (the Clapham Junction rail crash, the Piper Alpha explosion, the Barings Bank rogue trader, etc.). The long title of PIDA indeed indicates its intention: 'to protect individuals who make certain disclosures of information in the public interest; to allow such individuals to bring action in respect of victimisation; and for connected purposes.' The Public Interest Disclosure Act 1998 introduced legal protection for individuals who disclose information to expose acts such as criminal acts. The equivalent legislation in Northern Ireland is the Public Interest Disclosure (Northern Ireland) Order 1998. The legislation made substantial amendments to the Employment Rights Act 1996 (ERA) – and the Employment Rights (NI) Order 1996 in Northern Ireland – to protect whistleblowers in certain circumstances from dismissal and detrimental treatment by their employer. In some cases, whistleblowers may bring a case before an employment tribunal, which can award compensation.

Whistleblowing claims raise two basic questions. First, did the claimant make a protected disclosure? Second, if so, was the protected disclosure the cause of the claimant's dismissal, or some other detriment suffered by the claimant?

Auld LJ, in **Street v. Derbyshire Unemployed Workers Centre** [2005] ICR 97, significantly emphasised that:

> the purpose of the 'whistleblowing' provisions in the 1996 Act is *to encourage and protect employees to, and who, report concerns about malpractice in the workplace and elsewhere.* [Cited in para. 59, Sally Robertson Cloisters (2011).] [emphasis added]

However, he also warned that the purpose of the legislation was not to allow persons to advance personal grudges 'to advance personal antagonism' (see court report [2004] ICR 213, para. 30).

Whistleblowers are generally discouraged, despite their enormous courage. Firstly, many workers are faced with an anti-whistleblowing culture in the workplace, and

PIDA may only have limited efficacy in displacing this. Secondly, PIDA's provisions do provide a useful guideline on protected disclosures. Thirdly, the benefits to society which accrue from whistleblowing must be reflected in the protections offered by PIDA. The strict legal requirements posited by PIDA may be too harsh and costly compared to the benefits accrued in reality. Fourthly, the recourse offered by PIDA in the face of reprisals is inadequate. Whistleblowers are neither protected from reprisals before disclosures have been made nor after dismissal from discrimination during the job search process. Lastly, PIDA is silent on the burden of proof. This evasive stance leads to uncertainty and possibly formidable conditions.

The Health Service Circular 1999/198 states that every National Health Service (NHS) trust and health authority should have in place policies and procedures which comply with the Public Interest Disclosure Act and, as a minimum, include:

- guidance to help staff who have concerns about malpractice raise these reasonably and responsibly with the right parties
- the designation of a senior manager or non-executive director with specific responsibility for addressing concerns which need to be handled outside the usual management chain
- a clear commitment that staff concerns will be taken seriously and investigated
- an unequivocal guarantee that staff who raise concerns responsibly and reasonably will be protected against victimisation.

The absence of a statutory 'public interest' test was compounded by the EAT's decision in Parkins v Sodexho Ltd [2002] that an employee can make a protected disclosure about a past, current or putative breach of his own contract of employment, even though such a disclosure may have nothing to do with the public interest. Parkins arguably paved the way for claims by bankers that they had been victimised for complaining that their own bonuses were too low.

Difficulties in taking action commonly include: a reluctance to speak directly in criticism; fear of retaliation, whether personal or organisational uncertainty about who else to refer to; an unwillingness to get a colleague into trouble; and the possibility of actionable legal claims under the tort of defamation. These difficulties are, arguably, compounded when there is a considerable power differential, for example seniority, there is a culture of collusion, or your job is not secure. However, it is argued that your duty to put patients' or service users' interests first and act to protect them must override any personal and professional loyalties. The Public Interest Disclosure Act 1998 provides legal protection against victimisation or dismissal for individuals who disclose information in order to raise genuine concerns and expose malpractice in the workplace.

The concept of 'truth' has emerged as a key problem in the practice of whistleblowing, where certain truths that are of public interest are actively censored within organisations (Contu, 2014; Miceli and Near, 2002; Weiskopf and Willmott, 2013). If employees face few or no ramifications for whistleblowing actions, employees are more likely to make spurious information public – maybe because they misunderstand the actions they think they have observed, misinterpret what counts as unacceptable risk, or perhaps even because they have malicious intent towards an employer (MacDougall, 2016). Existing research has demonstrated that whistle-blowing is an important mechanism for employee 'voice' when other internal chan-nels for addressing organisational wrongdoing have failed (for excellent review papers, see Dasguopta and Kesharwami, 2010; Near and Miceli, 1996; Winfield, 1990). Complaints made to the ombudsman over care funding are now said to have doubled in only five years. Plans to encourage people to save to meet their own social care costs in old age are being discussed. The majority of specialist nurses believe that the care provided to young people with mental health problems is inadequate and getting worse (Lees, 2016).

How adverse outcomes and complaints are managed may significantly impact on physician wellbeing and practice. A recent study aimed to investigate how depres-sion, anxiety and defensive medical practice were associated with doctors' actual and perceived support, the behaviour of colleagues and process issues regarding how complaints investigations are carried out. In the survey study, respondents were clas-sified into three groups: no complaint, recent/current complaint (within 6 months) or past complaint (Bourne et al., 2017). Each group completed specific surveys. British Medical Association (BMA) members were invited to complete an online survey – most felt supported by colleagues (61%), only 31% felt supported by management. Not following process (56%), protracted timescales (78%), vexatious complaints (49%), feeling bullied (39%) or victimised for whistleblowing (20%), and using complaints to undermine (31%) were reported. Perceived support by management, speaking to colleagues, fair/accurate documentation and being informed about rights, correlated positively with wellbeing and reduced defensive practice. Doctors worried most about professional humiliation following a complaint investigation (80%). Poor process, prolonged timescales and vexatious use of complaints systems are associated with decreased psychological welfare and increased defensive prac-tice. In contrast, perceived support from colleagues and management is associated with a reduction in these effects.

The act when an employee reports wrongdoing to someone who is able to stop it is often described as a process along a time-line that includes stages such as discovery or observation, evaluation, decision on whether to blow the whistle or not and some type of reaction to the whistleblowing (Bjørkelo et al., 2010). Negative consequences following whistleblowing (i.e. retaliation) can be defined as 'taking an undesirable action against a whistleblower – in direct response to the whistle-blowing – who reported wrongdoing internally or externally, outside the organisation' (Rehg et al., 2008: 222). Retaliation can be informal and unofficial (De Maria and Jan, 1997) and can take the form of, for instance, ostracism (Faulkner, 1998) or being treated as a 'leper' (Peters and Branch, 1972).

Traditional whistleblowing theories have suggested that whistleblowers engage first in a rational process in determining whether or not to blow the whistle on misconduct. Whistleblowing is an inherently stressful process; emotions and motivation might interfere to produce conscious and unconscious biases which impair the rationality of decision-making. The negative impact of these stressors on

whistleblowing may be made worse depending on who engages in the misconduct: a peer or an advisor. It is remarkable that much hostility that whistleblowers
receive comes from their peers. Mannion and Davies (2015) provide an interesting
discussion of this point. Only a third of doctors, they report, say their colleagues
supported their decision to speak out. Much retaliation has to do with fear. The
anthropologist Mary Douglas uses the term 'slimy' to capture the fear of one who
will not stay in his place, or rather, one whose place we do not even know. The
person is often what is most feared by organisations – individuals not functioning,
rather euphemistically, as 'team players'. As Charles Alford (2016) points out, 'The
language is banal, but the sentiment is primordial, reflecting the deepest fears of the
organisational man or woman'.

In a recent study, participants were presented with an ethical scenario where either a
peer or an advisor engages in misconduct, and the positive and negative consequences
of whistleblowing are either directed to the wrongdoer, department or university.
Participant responses to case questions were evaluated for whistleblowing intentions,
moral intensity, metacognitive reasoning strategies, and positive and negative, active
and passive emotions. Findings indicate that participants were less likely to report the
observed misconduct of an advisor as compared to a peer (McIntosh et al., 2017).

Recently, another famous whistleblower Edward Snowden, an employee of the US
National Security Agency's (NSA) defence contractor, disclosed the NSA's domestic
surveillance programme, claiming concerns over its effects on privacy, Internet freedom and basic civil liberties (Greenwald et al., 2013). US Federal prosecutors are
reportedly filing charges against Snowden for espionage, theft and conversion of government property (Finn and Horwitz, 2013), even though he is hailed as a hero in the
social media (Cohen, 2013). Whistleblowing is widely discussed in the context of politics and national security with recent high-profile cases of 'leaking' sensitive political
and military information to the internet for public scrutiny. The highest profile cases
are those of Julian Assange's WikiLeaks (with the strapline 'courage is contagious')
publishing Bradley Manning's (now 'Chelsea Manning' since a gender reassignment –
itself a bold form of moral courage) leak of US high-security information and
Edward Snowden's leak of classified information from the National Security Agency
(Rodulson et al., 2015). The impact of the political context on healthcare needs to
be understood, and is picked up in more detail in Chapter 6.

Individual whistleblowers may be perceived as 'heroes' by some (for champion-
ing patients' interests; for promoting better care; for challenging management)
but may be seen as villains by others (for stepping outside of usual processes;
for denigrating services; for damaging professional and organisational reputa-
tions) (Mannion and Davies, 2015). Indeed, within the literature and in the popular media, whistleblowers are often portrayed either as 'courageous employees',
who act to maintain standards at great personal cost, or as 'disloyal malcontents',
who 'snitch' or 'grass' on colleagues, and pursue their own interests regardless
of the dysfunctional consequences for individuals and organisations (Jones and
Kelly, 2014). The review by Near and Miceli (1996) of whistleblowing found that
whistleblowers often turn to external channels as a tactic to increase the chances
of their message being heard. In public debate, 'whistleblowers' are variously

portrayed as 'heroes' standing up against a morally corrupt system or as 'traitors' who threaten the moral integrity of this very same system (Grant, 2002).

The consequences for whistleblowers often include: economic hardship, family stress, divorce and even suicide (Webber, 1989). The retaliation methods with the greatest physiological effect are isolation and humiliation; the whistleblower may be prevented from having access to information, and have resources such as their computer or telephone taken away, while they are assigned duties such as sweeping the floor to diminish their dignity (Kaplan and Kleiner, 2000). Moore and McAuliffe (2012: 341) have suggested that 'in order to increase the level of reporting amongst nurses in Ireland we need to address the key factors that prohibit them reporting poor care. It is clear, then, that the retaliation have a huge spectrum of effects, but all sufficient to obliterate completely a mutual feeling of trust and confidence between parties in a working environment. Two most common beliefs and fears amongst non-reporters are both *'fear of retribution'* and *'wouldn't want to cause trouble'*, both of which need to be addressed (p. 341). The study also found that non-reporters believe that incidents of poor care should be raised anonymously, and have a desire for appropriate risk management structures and ethics committees to be in place. Addressing these issues is the first step in encouraging non-reporters to report. The need to consider both voice and silence in the round are proposed to be crucial in organisational settings (Mannion and Davies, 2015).

However, not all people who raise concerns face negative consequences and lessons need to be learnt from those discussed in Chapter 3 who, despite the high level of sensitivity of issues raised, managed to do so and secure a positive outcome.

Kerfoot (1999) describes how the culture of courage is linked to a culture of integrity. She suggests that from a patient's perspective, this is about being account-able for our actions and truthful about when we make mistakes, and about staff being accountable and truthful to each other when we have made a mistake or if we believe colleagues are not upholding the standards of the profession. Challenging this can prove difficult when you are working in close proximity and everyone else is turning a blind eye.

The fictional example from practice 5.2 below illustrates some of these issues.

Example from Practice 5.2

Helen, Junior Manager, District General Hospital

Helen, a junior manager in a busy District General Hospital, bumped into an anaesthe-tist who had just left the operating theatre. Looking distressed, she asked him what the matter was. He shared his frustration about a procedure that hadn't gone well and that he had no confidence in the surgeon operating. Helen asked some questions to establish exactly what he meant by that statement which the anaesthetist then elaborated on. Helen asked him what he wanted to do about these concerns and he responded saying, 'What can I do?' Helen offered a series of options in terms of looking at outcome data and speaking to the surgeon directly but the anaesthetist said he wasn't comfortable to do this and just wanted to get home, saying goodnight. As he walked off Helen felt extremely uncomfortable as she had been given information that potentially placed patients at risk. That night she couldn't get the conversation out of her head and so in the morning went to find the anaesthetist to share her concerns. He dismissed them saying he had just been tired and to ignore him. Helen said she didn't feel able to do that and wanted him to speak to the medical director, which he refused to do and said he would deny the conversation if anyone asked.

Helen wasn't fully aware of the dynamics in the wider surgical team but knew that this couldn't be left so told the anaesthetist she would be going to see the medical director herself. She said she would not say who had told her about the concerns but that concerns had been raised.

She spoke to the medical director who listened and agreed to look into the matter, which he did and there was a training intervention put in to the surgical team.

Being removed from the immediacy of the situation and the relationships, Helen was able to raise concerns that the anaesthetist felt unable to but, at the same time, Helen was keen to maintain her relationship with the anaesthetist including him knowing he could trust her both to take action as a manager and not to breach a confidence.

Thus, for Helen and the anaesthetist, sharing concerns with others, asking questions and using the authority of the medical director who she believed would take positive action, enabled a difficult issue to be dealt with in a constructive manner. This will be explored further in Chapter 6.

Human factors

As already introduced in this book, firstly in Chapter 1, 'human factors', often referred to as ergonomics, is an established scientific discipline used in many other safety-critical industries.

Human factors approaches underpin current patient safety and quality improvement science, offering an integrated, evidenced and coherent approach to patient safety, quality improvement and clinical excellence. The principles and practices of human factors focus on optimising human performance through a better understanding of the behaviour of individuals, their interactions with each other and with their environment. By acknowledging human limitations, human factors offers ways to minimise and mitigate human frailties, so reducing medical error and its consequences. The system-wide adoption of these concepts offers a unique opportunity to support cultural change and empower the NHS to put patient safety and clinical excellence at its heart.

The role of the media

Reporting to media is an alternative in the current era of freedom of journalism in the country. Media reacts to mishaps earlier and wakes up the legal authorities. Very often journalists blow the whistle on general public matters. Like most things the role of the media is a double-edged sword. It rightly provides an important role in holding public servants and institutions to account but, at the same time, poor journalism that seeks high sales can lead to dramatic and simplistic headlines at the expense of complex and highly sensitive coverage, making learning and improvement more difficult.

Moving forward

This chapter began with the CIPD 'Courage to challenge'. These principles for all organisations are especially, if not even more, relevant to the NHS and social care. The CIPD propose, sensibly, this approach

- Consults others for ideas, advice and direction when facing unusual problems.
- Works closely with others who are involved in and impacted by the issue, consulting for their views and involving them in developing the solution.
- Explores and takes account of both the organisation's political forces and personal standing in a debate.
- Skilfully navigates and copes effectively with organisation politics. Is sufficiently self-reliant to manage extended periods of isolation or unpopularity in order to do the right thing.

We further explore how employees of the NHS and social care can achieve the above without resorting to 'whistleblowing' in Chapter 6, but this topic might require one book in itself. It is worth noting, however, that the intensity required in the 'courage to challenge' depends entirely on how hostile is the environment a person finds himself or herself in.

Useful Weblinks

www.england.nhs.uk/wp-content/uploads/2016/09/voicing-concerns-staff-policy.pdf
www.telegraph.co.uk/news/health/9177143/The-toxic-treatment-of-Dr-Drew.html

www.thetimes.co.uk/article/i-was-blacklisted-for-speaking-out-claims-nhs-whistleblower-l8g3hg8cpzp
http://blog.legalsolutions.thomsonreuters.com/legal-research/today-in-1912-the-lloyd-la-follette-act-was-enacted
http://swarb.co.uk/parkins-v-sodexho-ltd-eat-22-jun-2001
www.england.nhs.uk/wp-content/uploads/2013/11/nqb-hum-fact-concord.pdf
www.cipd.co.uk/Images/Courage-to-Challenge_tcm18-9692.pdf

References

Alford, C.F. (1999) 'Whistleblowers: How much we can learn from them depends on how much we can give up', *American Behavioral Scientist*, 43: 264–277.

Alford, C.F. (2001) *Whistleblowers: Broken Lives and Organisational Power*. Ithaca, NY: Cornell University Press.

Alford, C.F. (2016) 'What makes whistleblowers so threatening? Comment on "Cultures of Silence and Cultures of Voice: The Role of Whistleblowing in Healthcare Organisations", *International Journal of Health Policy and Management*, 5(1): 71–73.

Armstrong, A. and Francis, R.D. (2014) 'Legislating to protect the whistleblower: The Victorian experience', *The Australian Journal of Corporate Law*, 29: 101–111.

Auld L.J. (2005) Street v. Derbyshire Unemployed Workers Centre. ICR 97.

Aultman, J. (2008) 'Moral courage through a collective voice', *American Journal of Bioethics*, 8(4): 67–69.

BBC News (2016) 'Raj Mattu case: Sacked doctor gets £1.22m in damages', *BBC News*, 4 February. Available at: www.nytimes.com/2016/03/15/business/energy-environment/vw-diesel-emissions-scandal-whistleblower.html?_r=1 (accessed 6 June 2018).

Bjørkelo, B., Matthiesen, S.B. and Einarsen, S. (2010) 'Predicting proactive behaviour at work: Exploring the role of personality as an antecedent of whistleblowing behaviour', *Journal of Occupational and Organisational Psychology*, 83: 371–394.

BMJ (2016) 'Stephen Bolsin: Whistleblower on the Bristol scandal', *BMJ*, 352: i1328. Available at: www.bmj.com/content/352/bmj.i1328 (accessed 6 June 2018).

Bourne, T., De Cock, B., Wynants, L., Peters, M., Van Audenhove, C., Timmerman, D., Van Calster, B. and Jalmbrant, M. (2017) 'Doctors' perception of support and the processes involved in complaints investigations and how these relate to welfare and defensive practice: A cross-sectional survey of the UK physicians', *BMJ Open*, 7(11): e017856.

Bowden, P. (2014) *In the Public Interest: Protecting Whistleblowers and Those Who Speak Out*. Prahran, Victoria: Tilde.

Bradbury-Jones, C., Sambrook, S. and Irvine, F. (2007) 'The meaning of empowerment for nursing students: A critical incident study', *Journal of Advanced Nursing*, 59(4): 342–351.

Braillon, A. and Bewley, S. (2015) 'Which whistleblower is more vulnerable: The Indian doctor or nurse?', *BMJ*, 350: h1687.

Braithwaite, J., Matsuyama, Y., Mannion, R. and Johnson, J. (2015) Healthcare Reform, *Quality and Safety: Perspectives, Partnerships and Prospects in 30 Countries*. Burlington, VAA: Ashgate.

Bruhn, J.G. (2009) 'The functionality of gray area ethics in organizations', *Journal of Business Ethics* 89: 205. Available at: https://doi.org/10.1007/s10551-008-9994-7 (accessed 6 June 2018).

Calvert, J. (2002) 'How to buy the Olympics', *Guardian Unlimited*, 6 January.

Care Quality Commission (2013) *Whistleblowing Guidance for Providers who are Registered with the Care Quality Commission*, November. Available at: www.cqc.org.uk/sites/default/files/documents/20131107_100495_v5_00_whistleblowing_guidance_for_providers_registered_with_cqc.pdf (accessed 6 June 2018).

Cassematis, P.G. and Wortley, R. (2013) 'Prediction of whistleblowing or non-reporting observation: The role of personal and situational factors', *Journal of Business Ethics*, 117(3): 615–634.

Cleary, S.R. and Doyle, K.E. (2016) 'Whistleblowing need not occur if internal voices are heard: From deaf effect to hearer courage. Comment on "Cultures of Silence and Cultures of Voice: The Role of Whistleblowing in Healthcare Organisations"', *International Journal of Health and Policy Management*, 5(1): 59–61.

Cleary, S. and Duke, M. (2017) 'Clinical governance breakdown: Australian cases of wilful blindness and whistleblowing', *Nursing Ethics*, December. Available at: www.nursingreview.com.au/2017/12/whistleblowing-what-leads-a-nurse-to-make-the-call (accessed 6 June 2018).

Cohen, J. (2013) 'Most Americans back NSA tracking phone records, prioritize probes over privacy', *The Washington Post*, 10 June. Available at: www.washingtonpost.com/politics/most-americans-support-nsa-tracking-phone-records-prioritize-investigations-over-privacy/2013/06/10/51e721d6-d204-11e2-9f1a-1a7cdee20287_story.html?noredirect=on&utm_term=.e231165f559a (accessed 6 June 2018).

Contu, A. (2014) 'Rationality and relationality in the process of whistleblowing: Recasting whistleblowing through readings of Antigone', *Journal of Management Inquiry*, 23(4): 393–406.

Cueller, M., Keil, M. and Johnson, R.D. (2006) 'An investigation of the deaf effect response to bad news reporting in information systems projects', Georgia State University. Available at: http://muse.jhu.edu/article/221684/pdf (accessed 10 May 2015).

Dasguopta, S. and Kesharwami, A. (2010) 'Whistleblowing: A survey of the literature', *The IUP Journal of Corporate Governance*, 9(4): 57–70.

De Maria, W. and Jan, C. (1997) 'Eating its own: The whistleblower's organisation in vendetta mode', *Australian Journal of Social Issues*, 32(1): 37–59.

Department of Health (2015) *Culture Change in the NHS: Applying the Lessons of the Francis Inquiries*. London: Department of Health. Available at: https://assets.publishing.service.gov.uk/government/uploads/system/uploads/attachment_data/file/403010/culture-change-nhs.pdf (accessed 6 June 2018).

Devine, T. (2012) 'Corporate whistleblowers gain new rights and opportunities in the US', *Space for Transparency* [Blog]. Available at: http://blog.transparency.org/2012/10/01/corporate-whistleblowers-gain-new-rights-and-opportunities-in-the-us/ (accessed 6 June 2018).

Drew, D. (2014) *Little Stories of Life and Death @NHSWhistleblowr*. Kinworth Beauchamp, Leicestershire: Matador Books.

Dungan, J., Waytz, A. and Young, L. (2015) 'The psychology of whistleblowing', *Current Opinion in Psychology*, 6: 129–133.

Dyer, C. (2015) 'Francis report recommends a whistleblowing guardian in every NHS organisation', *BMJ*, 350: h828.

Dyer, C. (2017) 'Whistleblowing junior doctor scores victory in Court of Appeal', *BMJ*, 357: j2235.

Ewing, J. (2016) 'VW whistleblower's suit accuses carmaker of deleting data', *New York Times*, 14 March. Available at: www.nytimes.com/2016/03/15/business/energy-environment/vw-diesel-emissions-scandal-whistleblower.html?_r=1 (accessed 6 June 2018).

Faulkner, S.L. (1998) 'After the whistle is blown: The aversive impact of ostracism', PhD thesis, University of Toledo, Toledo, OH.

Finn, P. and Horwitz, S. (2013) 'US charges Edward Snowden with espionage in leaks about NSA surveillance programs', *The Washington Post*, 21 June. Available at: www.washingtonpost.com/world/national-security/us-charges-snowden-with-espionage/2013/06/21/507497d8-dab1-11e2-a016-92547bf094cc_story.html?utm_term=.af66f2e7cdf8 (accessed 6 June 2018).

Firth-Cozens, J., Firth, R. and Booth, S. (2003) 'Attitudes to and experiences of reporting poor care', *Clinical Governance: An International Journal*, 8(4): 331–336.

Firtko, A. and Jackson, D. (2005) 'Do the ends justify the means? Nursing and the dilemma of whistleblowing', *Australian Journal of Advanced Nursing*, 23(1): 51–60.

Fletcher, J.J., Sorrell, J.M. and Silva, M.C. (1998) 'Whistleblowing as a failure of organisational ethics', *The Online Journal of Issues in Nursing*, 3(3).

Garzón, B, Bourdon, W. (2017) Rebels with a cause: Africa's whistleblowers need urgent protection, The Guardian, Fri 10 Mar 2017, https://www.theguardian.com/world/2017/mar/10/rebels-with-a-causeafricas-whistleblowers-need-urgent-protection (online, accessed 13 Sep 2018).

Giacalone, R.A. and Promislo, M.D. (2013) 'Broken when entering: The stigmatization of goodness and business ethics education', *Learning & Education*, 12(1): 86–101. Available at: https://journals.aom.org/doi/10.5465/amle.2011.0005A (accessed 6 June 2018).

Gino, F. and Bazerman, M.H. (2009) 'When misconduct goes unnoticed: The acceptability of gradual erosion in others' unethical behaviour', *Journal of Experimental Social Psychology*, 45: 708–719.

GMC (2014) *Good Medical Practice*. Available at: www.gmc-uk.org/ethical-guidance/ethical-guidance-for-doctors/good-medical-practice (accessed 28 April 2018).

Grant, C. (2002) 'Whistle blowers: Saints of secular culture', *Journal of Business Ethics*, 39: 391–399.

Grealish, L. and Trevitt, C. (2005) 'Developing a professional identity: Student nurses in the workplace', *Contemporary Nurse*, 19(1–2): 137–150.

Greenwald, G., MacAskill, E. and Poitras, L. (2013) 'Edward Snowden: The whistleblower behind the NSA surveillance revelations', *The Guardian*, 11 June. Available at: www.theguardian.com/world/2013/jun/09/edward-snowden-nsa-whistleblower-surveillance (accessed 6 June 2018).

Harris, H. (1999) 'Courage as a management virtue', *Business and Professional Ethics Journal*, 18(3/4): 27–46.

Hesselbein, F. (2005) 'The leaders we need', *Leader to Leader*, 35: 4–6.

Hilton, C. (2016) 'Whistle-blowing and duty of candour in the National Health Service: A "history and policy" case study of the 1960s and 2010s', *Journal of the Royal Society of Medicine*, 109(9): 327–330.

Holt, K. (2015) 'Whistleblowing in the NHS', *BMJ*, 350: h2300.

Huberts, L. (2014) *Integrity of Governance: What It Is, What We Know, What Is Done and Where To Go*. New York, NY: Palgrave Macmillan.

Iedema, R., Jorm, C., Wakefield, J., Ryan, C. and Dunn, S. (2009) 'Practising open disclosure: Clinical incident communication and systems improvement', *Sociology of Health and Illness*, 31(2): 262–277.

Jackson, D., Hickman, L.D., Hutchinson, M., Andrew, S., Smith, J., Potgieter, I., Cleary, M. and Peters, K. (2014) 'Whistleblowing: An integrative literature review of data-based studies involving nurses', *Contemporary Nurse*, 48(2): 240–252.

Jolliff, T. (2016) *We Must Change the Bullying Culture in the NHS*, 17 November [blogpost]. Available at: www.leadershipacademy.nhs.uk/blog/must-change-bullying-culture-nhs (accessed 11 June 2018).

Jones, A. (2015) 'The role of employee whistleblowing and raising concerns in an organisational learning culture – elusive and laudable? Comment on "Cultures of silence and cultures of voice: The role of whistleblowing in healthcare organisations"', *International Journal of Health Policy Management*, 5(1): 67–69.

Jones, A. and Kelly, D. (2014) 'Whistle-blowing and workplace culture in older people's care: Qualitative insights from the healthcare and social care workforce', *Sociology of Health and Illness*, 36: 986–1002.

Kälvemark, S., Höglund, A.T., Hansson, M.G., Westerholm, P. and Arnetz, B. (2004) 'Living with conflicts-ethical dilemmas and moral distress in the health care system', *Social Science & Medicine*, 58(6): 1075–1084.

Kaplan, B. and Kleiner, B.H. (2000) 'New developments concerning discrimination for whistleblowing', *Equal Opportunities International*, 19(6): 75–77.

Kerfoot, K. (1999) 'The culture of courage', *Nursing economic$*, 17(4): 238–239.

Killingsworth, S. (2012) 'Modeling the message: Communicating compliance through organisational values and culture', *Georgetown Journal of Legal Ethics*, 25(4). Available at: https://ssrn.com/abstract=2161076 (accessed 11 June 2018).

Lachman, V.D. (2007) 'Moral courage: A virtue in need of development?', *Medsurg Nursing*, 16(2): 131–133.

Lachman, V.D. (2010) 'Strategies necessary for moral courage', *OJIN*, 15(3). Available at: http://dx.doi.org/10.3912/OJIN.Vol15No03Man03 (accessed 11 June 2018).

Lees, G. (2016) 'Produce a positive strategy for whistleblowing', *Nursing Standard*, 31(8): 32.

Levett-Jones, T. and Lathlean, J. (2009) '"Don't rock the boat": Nursing students' experiences of conformity and compliance', *Nurse Education Today*, 29(3): 342–349.

Luk, L.A., Ng, W.A., Ko, K.K. and Ung, V.H. (2008) 'Nursing management of medication errors', *Nursing Ethics*, 15(1): 28–39.

MacDonald, D. (2002) *A Guide to Moral Decision Making*. Available at: www.ethicsweb.ca/guide (accessed 27 January 2008).

MacDougall, D.R. (2016) 'Whistleblowing: Don't encourage it, prevent it – comment on "Cultures of silence and cultures of voice: The role of whistleblowing in healthcare organisations"', *International Journal of Health Policy and Management*, 5(3): 189–191.

Mannion, R. and Davies, H.T. (2015) 'Cultures of silence and cultures of voice: The role of whistleblowing in healthcare organisations', *International Journal of Health Policy and Management*, 4(8): 503–505.

Mansbach, A., Ziedenberg, H. and Bachner, Y. (2012) 'Nursing students' willingness to blow the whistle', *Nurse Education Today*, 33(1).

Mayer, D.M. (2016) 'Why are some whistleblowers vilified and others celebrated?', 1 September, *Harvard Business Review*. Available at: https://hbr.org/2016/09/why-are-some-whistleblowers-vilified-and-others-celebrated (accessed 11 June 2018).

McDonald, S. and Ahern, K. (2000) 'The professional consequences of whistleblowing by nurses', *Journal of Professional Nursing*, 16(6): 313–321.

McIntosh, T., Higgs, C., Turner, M., Partlow, P., Steele, L., MacDougall, A.E., Connelly, S. and Mumford, M.D. (2017) 'To Whistleblow or Not to Whistleblow: Affective and Cognitive Differences in Reporting Peers and Advisors', *Science and Engineering Ethics*. doi: 10.1007/s11948-017-9974-3.

Meurier, C.E. (2000) 'Understanding the nature of errors in nursing: Using a model to analyse critical incident reports of errors', *Journal of Advanced Nursing*, 32(1): 202–207.

Miceli, M. and Near, J. (2002) 'What makes whistleblowers effective? Three field studies', *Human Relations*, 55(4): 455–479.

Mooney, H. (2011) 'NHS whistleblowers are still being gagged, warns Baby P doctor', *BMJ*, 343: d8202.

Moore, L. and McAuliffe, E. (2010) 'Is inadequate response to whistleblowing perpetuating a culture of silence in hospitals?', *Clinical Governance: An International Journal*, 15(3): 166–178.

Moore, L. and McAuliffe, E. (2012) 'To report or not to report? Why some nurses are reluctant to whistleblow', *Clinical Governance: An International Journal*, 17(4): 332–342. Available at: http://dx.doi.org/10.1108/14777271211273215 (accessed 11 June 2018).

Near, J. and Miceli, M. (1996) 'Whistleblowing: Myth and Reality', *Journal of Management*, 22(3): 507–526.

Needham, N. (2012) 'Whistleblowing – a dangerous choice? Medical students have a duty to report on substandard care', *Student BMJ*, 20(e7870): 14–16.

NHS England (2016) *Voicing Your Concerns for Staff (Whistleblowing Policy)*. Available at: www.england.nhs.uk/wp-content/uploads/2016/09/voicing-concerns-staff-policy.pdf (accessed 11 June 2018).

Pears, D. (2004) 'The Anatomy of Courage', *Social Research*, 71(1): 1–12.

Perlow, L. and Williams, S. (2003) 'Is silence killing your company?', *Harvard Business Review*, 81(5): 52–58, 128.

Perry, N. (1998) 'Indecent exposures: Theorizing whistleblowing', *Organisation Studies*, 19: 235–257.

Peters, C. and Branch, T. (1972) *Blowing the Whistle: Dissent in the Public Interest*. New York, NY: Praeger.

Press Association (2016) 'Dismissed NHS whistleblower who exposed safety concerns handed £1.22m', *The Guardian*, 4 February. Available at: www.theguardian.com/uk-news/2016/feb/04/dismissed-nhs-whistleblower-who-exposed-safety-concerns-handed-122m (accessed 11 June 2018).

Reason, J. (1998) 'Achieving a safe culture: Theory and practice', *Work & Stress*, 12(3): 293–306.

Reason, J. (2002) *The Human Contribution: Unsafe Acts, Accidents and Heroic Recoveries*. Farnham: Ashgate.

Rees, C.E., Monrouxe, L.V. and McDonald, L.A. (2015) '"My mentor kicked a dying woman's bed": Analysing UK nursing students' "most memorable" professionalism dilemmas', *Journal of Advanced Nursing*, 71(1): 169–180.

Rehg, M.T., Miceli, M.P., Near, J.P. and Van Scotter, J.R. (2008) 'Antecedents and outcomes of retaliation against whistleblowers: Gender differences and power relations', *Organisation Science*, 19(2): 221–240.

Rodulson, V., Marshall, R. and Bleakley, A. (2015) 'Whistleblowing in medicine and in Homer's *Iliad*', *Medical Humanities*, 6 May. Available at: http://mh.bmj.com/content/early/2015/05/06/medhum-2015-010673 (accessed 11 June 2018).

Runciman, W.B., Helps, S.C., Sexton, E.J. and Malpas, A.A. (1998) 'A classification for incidents and accidents in the healthcare system', *Journal of Nursing*, 97(11): 35–43.

Sally Robertson Cloisters (2011) 'All in good faith. Whistleblowing law and practice', Employment Law Association. 14 December 2011. Available at: https://www.cloisters.com/images/easyblog_images/45/sallyrobertsonwhistleblowingeladec11.pdf

Sellin, S.C. (1995) 'Out on a limb: A qualitative study of patient advocacy in institutional nursing', *Nursing Ethics*, 2(1): 19–29.

Shannon, S.E., Foglia, M.B., Hardy, M. and Gallagher, T.H. (2009) 'Disclosing errors to patients: Perspectives of registered nurses', *Joint Commission Journal on Quality and Patient Safety*, 35(1): 5–12.

Shoesmith, S. (2016) *Learning from Baby P*. London: Jessica Kingsley Publishers.

Snyder, C.R. and Lopez, S.J. (2002) *Handbook of Positive Psychology*. London: Oxford University Press.

Somers, M.J. and Casal, J.C. (1994) 'Organisational commitment and whistleblowing: A test of the reformer and the organisation man hypothesis', *Group and Organisation Management*, 19(3): 270–284.

Srivastva, S. and Cooperrider, D.L. (1998) *Organisational Wisdom and Executive Courage*. San Francisco, CA: The New Lexington Press.

Vandekerckhove, W. and Tsahuridu, E. E. (2010) 'Risky rescues and the duty to blow the whistle', *Journal of Business Ethics*, 97: 365–380.

Verschoor, C.C. (2003) 'Eight ethical traits of healthy organisation', *Strategic Finance*, 85(3): 20–30.

Verschoor, C.C. (2004) 'Toward a corporation with conscience', *Strategic Finance*, 85(7): 20.

Vincent, C., Stanhope, M.N. and Crowley-Murphy, M. (1999) 'Reasons for not reporting adverse incidents: An empirical study', *Journal of Evaluation in Clinical Practice*, 5(1): 13–21.

Wakefield, M. and Maddox, P. (2000) 'Patient quality and safety problems in the US: Challenges for nursing', *Nursing Economics*, 18: 58–66.

Watson, C.L. and O'Connor, T. (2017) 'Legislating for advocacy: The case of whistleblowing', *Nursing Ethics*, 24(3): 305–312.

Webber, R.A. (1989) 'Whistleblowing', *Executive Excellence*, 6(7): 9–10.

Weiskopf, R. and Willmott, H. (2013) 'Ethics as critical practice: The Pentagon papers, deciding responsibly, truth-telling, and the unsettling of organisational morality', *Organisation Studies*, 34: 469–494.

Winfield, M. (1990) *Minding Your Own Business: Self-regulation and Whistleblowing in British Companies*. London: Social Audit.

Wise, J. (2016) 'General practices must appoint whistleblowing guardian', *BMJ*, 355: i6266.

Wylie, C. (2018) 'Christopher Wylie: Why I broke the Facebook data story – and what should happen now', *The Guardian*, 7 April. Available at: www.theguardian.com/uk-news/2018/apr/07/christopher-wylie-why-i-broke-the-facebook-data-story-and-what-should-happen-now (accessed 11 June 2018).

COURAGE TO FLOURISH

REBECCA MYERS

Being deeply loved by someone gives you strength, while loving someone deeply gives you courage.

Lao Tzu

The chapter will consider how a more substantial re-thinking about healthcare systems might be needed, such as a less retributive approach to healthcare regulation and a more inclusive way of organising and providing healthcare that opens it up to more diverse views on what is happening and why, in order to promote organisational development and learning. We will try to bring together some of the themes which have emerged in our discussion of courage in this book. Fundamental to thinking about how courage can 'flourish' is the answer to the question: 'Under what professional, personal and environmental conditions should someone need to show courage and when does the need for courage suggest there is a problem?'

The chapter will also consider what can and is being done through different lenses, be it as individuals, teams, organisations or collectively as a wider society.

We have tried to define what courage is in Chapter 1, and why and when we think it should or should not be needed. We have explored different perspectives and examples of people stepping forward to lead and do courageous acts. All the cases have highlighted the wider context in which individuals act and the importance of understanding the dynamics of relationships. These relationships are influenced at multiple levels and thus increasing the conditions for the types of 'pro social' behaviours we would require in healthcare, we need to consider these at multiple levels.

A collective purpose

One of the core elements of finding ways for addressing the issues in this book is attempting to build a collective purpose.

As the NHS reaches its 70th birthday, it continues to occupy a unique place in public consciousness. However, it is under significant pressure and facing perhaps its biggest challenges since it was established. In a recent survey by Ipsos MORI of 1151 adults (aged 15 and over in England), 77% of the public believe the NHS should be maintained in its current form. This level of support has remained consistent over almost two decades despite widespread social, economic and political change. Around 90% of people support the founding principles of the NHS, indicating that these principles are just as relevant today as when the NHS was established.

The former Secretary of State for Health and Social Care, Jeremy Hunt MP, declared an ambition to make it 'the safest in the world', and has been praised for leadership globally in patient safety. This is a laudable aim and one that in its intention can unite those working in it, using it, funding it and being accountable for it. But to do that we need to create the environment in which, when required, people are able to undertake the courageous work to face the emotional and physical demands of illness and mortality and don't have to feel anxious or courageous in the need to speak up about any concerns or errors.

Individual contributions

In any effort to create change, we need to look at our own contribution to situations and to work with those things we can directly control or influence. Focusing on what we can directly control or influence can help us manage our frustration and risk of burnout as we become more proactive in our interactions and thus have a greater sense of choice and autonomy. Being intelligent about when, and how, to speak up to ensure maximum benefit to patients and the NHS whilst minimising risk to ourselves is a key part of being courageous.

Using a framework such as Covey's 'Circle of Control' (Covey, 1999) helps us to systematically work through what is within our sphere of influence and control, recognising areas which may require support from others who have different roles and spheres of influence. A 'Circle of Influence' encompasses those concerns that we can do something about. Stephen Covey describes our behaviour as a function of our decisions, rather than our conditions.

A framework can assist all of us to think through our approach to a situation and to work collectively to achieve a positive outcome. One of the challenges of using such a framework is being able to be realistic about what is within our control. As a coach one of the authors (RM) works with people to explore the individual's perception of their internal or external locus of control. Individuals have a predisposition to certain views, for example, I am responsible, capable, accountable for what happens (internal), or I am not responsible, capable, accountable (external). Being able to discuss with colleagues and trusted confidantes will help to get a realistic view to help determine how to approach a situation and what we can do ourselves and when we need others. Conversations with others is a critical starting point for addressing and resolving ethical problems, which enables health and social care professionals to take actions that require 'moral courage'.

It is important to appreciate that, irrespective of our actions, in complex systems we cannot control the outcomes, thus even with a specific intent we can never know the full impact of what we have done. This understanding of the inability to control outcomes can both free us up, or inhibit us to act as it also recognises the shared responsibility for events and responses to them rather than locating this solely with the individual. These types of interactions work more along the approach of the adult–adult interaction we explored in Chapter 2 (Berne, 1964).

Courage to do the work of healthcare – managing our own anxiety

As we have shown throughout, working in healthcare is inherently demanding emotionally and we are often faced with our own anxieties ('Do I know what I am doing?', 'Can I help this patient?', 'How do I manage my own distress?') as well as those around us – be it patients and their families or other colleagues. Being able to recognise our own signs of anxiety and using techniques to assist us can help us to focus our attention on what is required of us and what we need to do ourselves or seek assistance for.

As explored in Chapter 3, the courage required in clinical medicine is the 'reliable disposition to approach, with the appropriate level of confidence, situations that are fraught with the realistic fear of getting it wrong and causing harm as well as courage to competently discharge the inescapable obligations to decide and act despite the irreducible uncertainty' (Hamric et al., 2015).

Irrespective of skill and experience, health professionals can never totally control how patients will respond to illness and thus fully know whether the outcomes of their interventions, or their own abilities, are what helped or hindered the situation. It is important to remember that our responsibilities always outstrip our control and to maintain humility in our work. The stakes in healthcare are particularly high, the responsibility daunting, and resources often inadequate such that the practice of healthcare will never be free of the risks of insufficient information, imperfect reasoning and distracted attention. Insight into the state of our own health and wellbeing is vital, but if we are too burnt out or clinically unwell, we might be dangerously lacking this vital insight.

Political intelligence to facilitate courage

Whilst often seen as a negative aspect of organisational life, ignoring organisational politics can result in difficulties for individuals and their ability to meet the organisation's purpose. The skill is for individuals to understand organisational politics and then navigate it in a way that is constructive by aligning your behaviour to the organisation's purpose. In his book, *Workplace Politics* (Bancroft-Turner, 2008) suggests that there are four key skills of political intelligence:

- Communication – active listening and honesty
- Influencing – adopting a win–win outlook
- Networking – building alliances for common good
- 'Factor X' – understanding your power and using it in a generative manner.

Recognising these and developing strengths in these areas help individuals to find ways to speak out in a way that reduces the likelihood of negative consequences.

Power and love

> When nobody is talking about power, that is where it unquestionably exists, at once secure and great in its unquestionability.
>
> Ulrich Beck

Working effectively in any context requires an understanding of power, the different sources and how to use it effectively for the organisational purpose; whilst we may have positional power when in senior positions, we need to rely on those with 'expert' power to guide us. Personal power (e.g. charisma) can be needed for us to be effective in creating the right conditions for our work, thus appreciating at different times we will need to use or call upon others' different sources of power to get things done. Understanding your own sources and those of others around you is critical in knowing how to navigate difficult situations, which require you to challenge others, or direct requests. Far too often, people see power simply through a hierarchical lens and either feel unable to act as they are in a lower position in the formal hierarchy or have an aversion to those in hierarchy and look for methods to undermine them – neither being a successful strategy.

In an environment where quick and vital decisions need to be taken due to high-risk, complex and stressful situations, it is understandable that mistakes can be made. In this situation the ability to be confident to speak up when a potential error is happening and to have the humility to know that, even with significant training and experience, you make mistakes, is critical. But speaking up is only the start of our work and we must act on 'truth' and support others when they speak and act on their truth against the misuse of power by those in authority, thus creating the conditions within us to speak out in the interest of the wider whole rather than just our own position.

Ira Chaleff (2015) asks us to work hard at maintaining both personal freedom and accountability (power) and social cohesion (love) but to do this not in blind resistance or acceptance to authority or cohesion but through '*intelligent disobedience*' that incorporates the values and practice of personal accountability. Chaleff interestingly borrows the phrase 'intelligent disobedience' from the field of guide dog training, where it refers to a quality that trainers seek to instil in guide dogs. The fact that guide dogs must be trained to obey commands is obvious. What may not be so obvious is that they must also be trained to disobey commands. These practices act as protection for both the individual and the interests of the group. But challenging someone not acting in line with the wider purpose or values, or when a new way of seeing needs to be proposed, can require people to step out alone (Brown, 2017). People who are able to stand apart from the crowd and question or critique others' views and behaviours can often find themselves alone. With human beings having an inherent need for belonging, this can be a difficult and lonely place. It requires people to be able to standalone but also to continue to have an open mind and compassion towards those who we fundamentally disagree with.

Part of what can help us to standalone includes setting clear boundaries, and holding and respecting them. It requires us to let go of being liked by everyone or worrying about disappointing people. We need to be reliable and say what we mean and mean what we say, including being open to saying when we have changed what we think and why. We need to be accountable and step forward when needed, taking responsibility for our own actions and not blaming others. We need to have integrity and practise our values even when they are tested or when we feel discomfort to be courageous enough to act and we need to be willing to see good in others and be generous in our assumptions of them.

Finally, as we have discussed in earlier chapters, we need to be able to be vulnerable, not to be consumed or taken advantage of, but to see it as a strength, not a weakness and the place where our 'brave self' steps forward (Brown, 2017).

Examining our own relationship with authority

Examining our own relationship to authority is important and being able to develop a 'healthy' attitude, which respects the position but is not unquestionably deferential, is important. An unhealthy relationship to perceived authority figures is one where there is deference to hierarchy versus expertise or moral code. Our attitude to authority often develops at an early age through experience of our first authority figures – parents and teachers. These relationships lead to a way of relating which often becomes habitual and is often not re-examined as we get older, becoming almost an automatic reflex. Being able to step back and reflect on our own patterns of relating enables us to see how effective they are both for us as individuals and for the wider organisational purpose.

In organisations that have strong hierarchical structure(s), such as the NHS, 'obedience' can get privileged over the higher-level skill of discerning when it's not right to obey. A hierarchical culture reinforces this, making a questioning of authority or failure to follow a request/command by someone in authority more difficult.

Example from Practice 6.1

Nicola, staff nurse

Nicola was the staff nurse who whilst on a night shift was instructed to administer some medication which she questioned the dosage of with the junior doctor. The doctor shouted at Nicola to give the drug and not to question his authority. When she showed him the dosage in the British National Formulary (BNF) he again dismissed her, saying he knew what the dosage should be for this patient and thus she must give it. With reluctance she administered the medication and documented what had happened. When she reported the incident afterwards, the night sister immediately suspended her for committing a drug error and she was given a written warning. When asked what had happened to the doctor in question, staff were told he had been 'spoken to by his consultant'. The patient in question was not unduly harmed but the nurse on return to work had lost her confidence and subsequently gave up nursing, as she felt unsupported. The story became well known amongst nursing staff on the ward and reinforced a message about what happens if you obey an order which you don't think is correct.

Reflections on Nicola's experience: A more effective approach, arguably, could have been for the nurse to have said to the doctor she had been taught that this dosage was harmful to the patient and so could not administer it, but that she had prepared the medication which he could give directly if he felt the dosage was accurate.

When looking at what conditions are present for healthcare providers to be willing to take action, this includes: recognising an issue as ethically problematic; believing the repercussions of one's actions can be handled; and a belief that positive changes will occur as a result of one's efforts (Cook and Hoas, 2008). We saw this in Stephanie's and Helen's case in Chapter 5.

Changing our way of relating

What can we do to help encourage people to raise concerns? How do we help individuals to know when to follow orders and when to question or challenge them?

Part of this is about being explicit in training for the need for this to occur. The World Health Organisation (2012) (WHO) has training programmes that explore with health professionals when to speak up and how to do so in a way that enables colleagues (in particular authority figures) to not become defensive or punitive in their response but be grateful for the challenge or pointing out of a potential error. This sits very much with the thinking of the WHO surgical safety checklist (2009), which aims to change the way the theatre team interacts through acknowledging the risks of hierarchy or hubris in surgical procedures.

When thinking about challenging authority it is also important to consider cultural influences. Some cultures place higher value on deference to authority than others. The more this is in place, the greater the need to ensure subordinates don't simply default to silence in high-risk situations to avoid those with authority losing face. What can assist in these situations is using 'mitigating language' when raising concerns which is less threatening and is somewhat deferential to reduce the perceived challenge to another's authority, especially if they are concerned with hierarchy; this could mean posing a question to raise a concern rather than a direct challenge. All too often, our way of relating has been about debate or adversarial in nature, based on a win–lose approach. This has been the dominant discourse for centuries and still features heavily in the education system through structures such as debating societies. We need to find other ways to relate to each other if we are to create different outcomes.

In his book, *Power and Love: A Theory and Practice of Social Change* (2010), Adam Kahane offers a way of negotiating some of our toughest challenges in society. He proposes that to date our approach to addressing our most difficult challenges has been at the edge of two extremes – the medium of aggressive wars or submissive peace, leaving us with a feeling of pain, resentment and feeling stuck. He advocates that to co-create new realities we need to work with two distinct fundamental forces that are in tension – power and love. The theologian and philosopher Paul Tillich (1886–1965) describes power as the 'drive of everything living to realise itself, with increasing intensity and extensity', thus making power the force in which one achieves their purpose, growth and gets their work done; similarly he defines love as 'the drive towards unity of the separated', thus love is the force to reconnect and make whole that which is seen to have fragmented (1954: 25, 36).

By recognising our interdependency this highlights the essential need for cooperation in our dealings with each other. Power and love have two sides, which are both generative and degenerative and are balanced by the use of the other. Thus 'power without love, can be reckless and abusive and love without power, can be sentimental and anaemic' (Kahane, 2010: 29–30).

Power in its generative form is about realising one's potential, and the degenerative side is about the suppression of another's potential. In a culture that constantly promotes a sense of 'self', we run the risk of ignoring the sense of 'other' which in turn can lead to a culture of fear and conflict. We need to be aware of how we are 'being' in relationship with others and constantly adjusting our behaviour in the service of making a positive difference. We see this in the case study of Philippa (described in Chapter 3) where she is trying to adjust her approach to support her colleague but also assert her position.

This awareness of how we are behaving needs to also consider the historical context in which we operate. In an attempt to change the hierarchical relationships that exist between different staff groups, patients and even gender and ethnicity, those who have traditionally held power over others often talk about how they need to 'empower' other people. This paradoxically continues the approach of 'power over' as they are seen as the people who will 'fix' the relationship dynamics. This is a common pattern seen in healthcare and is being challenged by a movement in 'patient leaders' (see work developed by David Gilbert and Mark Doughty on 'patient leaders' for example, Gilbert, (2014)). The challenge is for individuals to both own their power and know when to cede it in the service of the wider purpose.

Courage as a skill in taking 'calculated risks'

So can we teach people how to be courageous? If we understand the contributory factors that enabled those who have acted before, we can deconstruct the different elements and educate those in health and social care to adopt a similar approach.

As discussed in Chapter 1, courage and taking risks is a relative act based on a set of calculations. All of these calculations require an interaction with others and the wider context in which people are operating. Failure to recognise and acknowledge this perpetuates the appearance of the single individual who is or isn't courageous. This in turn places a significant burden on individuals to take action and, in response, to take total responsibility and accountability for the decisions. In an increasingly complex and challenging environment in healthcare, this can make the position of leadership or moral action less attractive, leading to people not wishing to step forward.

Successful leaders, demonstrating courage, will take carefully calculated risks, while accepting that failure can be an unfortunate by-product of success and innovation. In *Learning to Take Risks, Learning to Succeed*, published by NIESR in June 2010, the author Heather Rolfe argues that, 'Risk taking is essential to innovation: anyone developing a new product, service or idea risks the possibility that it will not work, that someone else will get there first or it will be met with disinterest'. In relation to innovation in the NHS, Neil Guha (2018), writing for The King's Fund blog, notes that, 'Ring-fenced time, autonomy, contributing to career progression and active encouragement to take calculated risk (at an individual and organisational level) are strong levers but I am not sure these are employed in a coherent or consistent manner.'

Taking calculated risks requires us to do our homework in understanding the issues we are facing as much as we can and raising issues in a way that is not threatening or accusatory to others without us understanding the full facts. It is easy to take the 'moral' high ground but, as seen in Chapter 3, the evidence suggests that how we think we would react in situations is not an accurate predictor of what we would really do.

Having 'difficult conversations'

As we have discussed previously in this book (Chapter 2), part of what is needed to be courageous is the ability to have difficult conversations.

Being able to negotiate and have 'difficult conversations' is key in healthcare, be it by health professionals breaking bad news to patients, telling their families they are ill or dying, to discussing the allocation of resources. Having a structure in which to do this can help. In order for courage to flourish, we need to get better at having 'difficult' conversations, be it with our colleagues, or with people using the NHS, politicians or the media. By having them, it will enable us to talk about our different perspectives and find ways to learn and change our approach to get better outcomes.

We can do this by: making it safe to talk – allow people to really share what they think and feel; listening from a place of curiosity not judgement; looking to build on each other's contributions rather than dismissing them; recognising the 'stories' in our heads and separating impact and intent; using the first person in our communications to take ownership of our own feelings and thoughts; and focusing on contribution and not blame, recognising we all contribute in some way. In addition, developing our skills in managing conflict and disagreement will assist us and the wider system (see Thomas Kilmann's Conflict Inventory as a useful framework to adopt). Like most things, adopting this takes time, practice and self-reflection, but building it into the training of those that work in healthcare and using it as a strategy for conversations with families who have concerns may enable more honest and productive conversations.

Developing our inquiry skills

A way to counter jumping to conclusions is to develop our skills in inquiry (Schein, 2013) and to hold a position of curiosity rather than rushing to judgement and to be aware of our own prejudices and assumptions. Finding ways to ask genuine questions around what people are doing and why, and being open to listening to diverse perspectives offer us insight into the world of the 'other' and an opportunity to find ways to work together to meet the shared purpose.

The relationship between 'self' and 'group'

> Moral courage takes place in the context of a community where words and ideas matter, where the individual rubs up against the collective expressions of humanity. (Kidder, 2006: 218)

As healthcare is a team activity, it is important to see the role of courage in the context of the group and in ways to support the development of high-performing teams.

Emotions and behavioural patterns which are observed in individual members, are often a phenomenon of the group but are located in one member. The need to understand the role of group dynamics and how to work effectively with these issues is important (see Bion's 1998 work in the 'Basic Assumption Group'). This usually manifests itself in people being seen as performing a particular function on behalf of the group such as the 'kind' one, the 'critical' one, etc. Failure to recognise this process can lead to people being labelled and others not taking their responsibility for performing a necessary group function.

So we start to see the wider social influences, and the individual 'in relation to' rather than as an independent actor. Our interpretations of their acts of courage are socially constructed and influenced by our own set of values and beliefs about what they do and why, as well as our knowledge of the wider context in which their acts took place (see Gergen's [1999] work on social constructionism).

By looking at courage through a group lens it gives us different insights into why and how things occur, and offers us different ways of 'being' with others. Understanding that we are not independent of our individual and social context, and that situations can be seen as fearful by some and not others, gives us choices about how to respond to situations that we believe need to be questioned and challenged, even if doing so creates anxiety or fear within us.

When looking at some of the underlying dimensions of human existence and how people behave, the concept of 'agency' and 'communion' is a helpful framework (Bakan, 1966). Agency represents a focus on the individual, striving for personal growth and promotion potentially as a way to pursue social dominance. Communion represents a focus upon others striving for contact and connection as a desire to preserve social bonds. When looked at from an evolutionary perspective, agency and communion define the behaviour and problems of group living which our ancestors had to adapt to and which all of us have to manage in modern-day society. Group living/working requires us to compete for resources, position, recognition, etc. (*agency*) whilst also cooperating to acquire resources, position, etc. as part of reciprocal alliances (*communion*).

Most of us are constantly balancing these different dimensions in order to manage relationships and our own needs.

This brings us back to the issue of social identity theory, and how strongly one attaches oneself to that group to feel able to speak out against it for fear of rejection. The role of the individual, relative to the authority of the group, is one that has existed since the beginning of time and there is always a tension. This tension needs to be constantly balanced such that if an individual is totally dismissive of authority then a culture cannot maintain itself or operate in a way that protects the rights of other individuals, and at the same time if the authority of the group is dismissive of the individual it dehumanises the culture it is charged with serving. What is required is to build into the culture the values and approaches that preserve the individual's freedom against the negative forces of conformity and obedience that it can generate. With the increased advent of social media and technology, individuals are able to be monitored and scrutinised, which can run the risk of compromising this approach and, at the same time, this technology can be used to help individuals join with like-minded people and organise themselves to counter negative pressure.

Much work has been done looking at what enables high performance in teams and specifically within the NHS, with 'real' teams being defined as those that have clear objectives, interdependent working and regular meetings to discuss effectiveness (West and Markiewicz, 2004). Unfortunately, many working in the NHS are in 'pseudo' teams reporting high levels of errors, accidents and poor staff wellbeing (West et al., 2012) and this in turn impacts on staff health and acts as a barrier to the provision of patient satisfaction and mortality rates (West and Dawson, 2012). Alongside the dynamic of the team is the role that the team leader plays, as referred to previously. Creating the right conditions at the team level is critical to creating the right conditions for staff to not feel fearful or need courage to speak up about concerns. Developing structures and processes that facilitate effective team working is key.

As we explored in Chapter 3, leadership is a social 'process' rather than simply the characteristics of individuals and needs to be seen in the context of people's relationships with those they work with and the context in which they are operating. Enabling people to know when to lead and when to follow is important for everyone. Seeking out regular feedback and finding 'courageous' followers will keep leaders and their organisations safe even if at times uncomfortable. In addition, when we are working with leaders we need to play our part in being courageous followers, not placing them on pedestals or abdicating our own responsibility in tackling issues – the work we do in healthcare is too important to simply leave it to someone else.

Organisational level

We also need to consider the position from an organisational perspective. Kilmann and colleagues (2011) developed a framework that identified four types of organisational experiences with courage against a matrix of high or low accounts of fear around performing acts of courage and high or low frequency of observed acts of possible courage. From this assessment they identified four types of organisations:

1. *The courageous organisation* – identified by members who observe potential acts of courage that can subsequently be defined as actual acts of courage because these acts take place despite fear.
2. *The fearful organisation* – identified by members who are overcome by the fear of being harmed and do not act.
3. *The bureaucratic organisation* – identified by members who neither observe acts of courage nor fear being harmed; they are resigned to following rules.
4. *The quantum organisation* – identified by members who either observe potential acts of courage (but not actual as fear is not present) or believe such acts are not needed because their organisation already supports doing what is in the best interest of key stakeholders.

This framework also shows the climate of the organisation in the context of a number of contributory factors that support or discourage organisational members from making positive contributions to the overall measures of performance and staff satisfaction, which include the experience of the external environment, the internal climate and culture, and the formal and informal systems which determine structures and people's roles.

Using a questionnaire such as this would enable organisational leaders to understand how they, and staff in it, currently view the organisation or their local team, creating an opportunity to look at what can be shared from those who are operating in a 'quantum' manner and what needs to shift for those operating in a 'fearful' organisation. The framework is helpful because it recognises that in a bureaucracy that is governed by rules and procedures as the tasks and processes are relatively simple and clear and do not need much discussion, there is little need for courage to do the work, but as the work in itself becomes more complex and there is less certainty then the need for staff to constantly review what happens and speak up when things are not going well is critical.

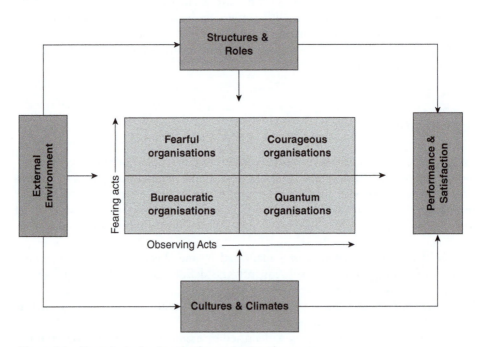

Figure 6.1   Nomological network of organisational courage

Source: Adapted from Kilmann et al. (2011)

For health and social care organisations and in particular the learning from those who have cited local leaders as the cause of the need to whistleblow, this highlights the influence of the external environment on the internal culture.

Courage is 'contagious'

Courage can be contagious and lead to a 'domino' effect of others acting too. We see this playing out in all areas of life such as the recent Twitter #MeToo campaign for women who have been affected by sexual harassment or discrimination to highlight their own experiences following the case against the allegations (as yet unproven) against Hollywood producer, Harvey Weinstein, or in cases of history of people like Rosa Parks who refused to stand up on a bus, leading to a shift by the civil rights movement and racial prejudice.

Moving into looking at courage from an organisational perspective, it is important to look at the context of providing healthcare. There has been a huge shift in work design for healthcare which is testing the resolve and intrinsic motivation of healthcare professionals for their work. Increased levels of demand, reduced levels of support, as everyone feels the pressure, and the ability to control work and the environment in which we operate, create an imbalance which can affect people's wellbeing. In order for staff to not only combat these changes but also to thrive and be able to continue to raise concerns and admit errors, they need to be supported and effective psychological interventions are key. In order for people to learn and grown they need to feel psychologically 'safe'. A key way to do that is through building strong and supportive attachments that reduce our anxiety; relationships that make us feel confident, competent and reassured (Bowlby, 1988).

In the context of healthcare, as we saw in the case study of Helen and the anaesthetist in Chapter 5, staff can feel unsure where to form these attachments, feeling a divided loyalty to the organisation, immediate colleagues, professional groups or to patients. Managers have the potential to assist staff in these difficulties, yet NHS managers are one of the most highly stressed occupational groups in the UK (Williams et al., 1999). In order for managers to help staff feel emotionally contained they need to be adequately contained themselves and so increased pressure on the managerial agenda, such as constant reorganisations, affects managers, staff and patients alike. The NHS has had at least 12 structural reorganisations in 26 years; Britnell's *In search of the Perfect Health System* (2015) speaks to this trend directly. Being willing to voice their own distress as managers can be difficult due to a perception that they 'should' be able to deal with this, 'that their work isn't as difficult as those doing the "real" work' and the negativity that those in management often face as being unnecessary burdens and a cost on healthcare.

Recognising that it is important to create conditions where all staff are able to be supported and have good connections, the use of reflective spaces such as Schwartz Center Rounds ® and action learning sets (described in Chapter 2) is key.

Organisational design

Paying attention to the design of work to reduce the need to be courageous is important. It requires regular review by managers who are appropriately trained and are skilful in this work and who are supported themselves by those in senior positions and leadership roles. Using the expertise of workforce teams and psychologically trained professionals to monitor, review and design organisational interventions offers an important approach to responding effectively to the wider context of individual staff.

A key part of enabling courage, when required, to flourish and to minimise the need for it to be required, is to build in strategies to the organisational design. In the frequent reification of organisations it can be easy to forget that the way we organise is (to a large extent) within our control and influence, and whilst we cannot control the outcomes we can be more or less thoughtful in being clear about our intentions and what may increase the likelihood of things occurring. Having organisational psychologists on site to recognise the trauma and be able to respond accordingly with evidence-based interventions is important and something the NHS still remains surprisingly poor at. In her book *Tales of Organisational Life*, Wren (2016) shares her experiences as an occupational psychologist working with staff on the impact of the nature of delivering healthcare in a London teaching hospital and the associated benefits staff reported from using the service.

We would argue that more attention needs to be paid to how the design of the work, the physical space in which it takes place, and the interactions with the technology used to deliver, monitor and improve care, create adverse conditions which then need staff to be courageous. Making data more accessible and to a diverse audience offers the opportunity for wider visibility and questioning of data and the ability to reduce the risk of groupthink (Janis, 1982), which may not see errors or risks due to a normalisation process. When staff are overwhelmed, their ability to see risk or poor practice can be affected, thus having those slightly removed who recognise staff's pressures and see their role as keeping everyone safe, is important.

Example from Practice 6.2

Risk assessment

An exercise with consultants and non-executive directors in a university teaching hospital asked them to review the risk and likelihood of a situation occurring from a series of case studies. The exercise revealed the two groups were at opposite ends of the spectrum around assessment of risk and impact and thus couldn't agree on what to report and what mitigation plans were required. Through this process there was a reassessment to enable both groups to agree on an approach that modified both extremes by using data and action plans to report to the sub-committee of the board which all felt was balanced and appropriate.

Efforts by organisations to display data on public websites or on ward boards enables discussion with patients and families, as well as external parties, to be open about performance but also to highlight to others the risk so they can participate in contributing to reductions through their own actions (for example, the 'Hospital Washing Hands Campaign'). Failure to address work design principles which marry the technical and social factors of organisational life limits opportunity for creating working environments that maximise the expertise of staff providing care, and continues to create risky conditions that mean staff are more likely to make errors and locate them within the individual rather than the wider system (Clegg et al., 2014). This applies not just to within organisations but also across them where visibility of data and decisions of the wider multidisciplinary team create opportunities to pick up any errors or check decisions to change things prior to implementation within a wider context of the individual's or system of care's performance.

Creating a learning organisation

Davies and Nutley's (2000) paper argued in the *BMJ* that building a learning organisation in the NHS requires attention to some key cultural values which include: celebration of success, absence of complacency, tolerance of mistakes, belief in human potential, recognition of tacit knowledge, openness, trust and being outward looking.

Creating a learning culture requires staff to be able to change their behaviours upon a deepening and broadening of their skills, knowledge and worldviews and that the role of leadership is to address the barriers that inhibit this. This includes the use of formal (structured learning programmes and developmental supervision) and informal (everyday working practices with time for questioning and reflection) learning opportunities. There is an important need to develop skills in those with managerial and leadership positions to be able to coach staff, contain their own anxiety and understand psychological processes that enhance all staff wellbeing and psychological safety to create a climate of fairness, open communication and empowerment.

Explicit reference to the risk of not challenging each other needs to be part of organisational life. Hermann Hospital in Texas introduce staff to the 'authority gradient' concept which draws everyone's attention to people's reluctance to challenge anyone they see as more senior or powerful and the associated risks (Turnball, 2001). They hand out cards which explain the concept and include the statement, ' I'm a team member and I have something important to say'. This is followed up by a clear commitment that staff will always be supported when questioning authority – thus creating a culture where courageous acts are not only encouraged but also expected. This message is also reinforced at awards and in newsletters where people who have spoken up are publicly recognised and thanked for doing so. This approach starts to shift the perception that speaking up and questioning is something to be feared to one that says it is normal, expected and valued.

Role of good governance

Understanding human relationships and how they affect behaviour is important but that alone cannot be used to create the conditions for courage. Whilst often criticised as bureaucratic and overly burdensome, governance structures can help to build in systems and processes that mean areas of risk or poor performance are constantly reviewed, minimising the need for people to 'speak out'. Dashboards that look at meaningful data around outcomes, and patient and staff experiences should act as early warning signs for leaders and enable them to focus support in areas where there are difficulties. The development of patient feedback sites such as 'Care Opinion' are offering ways for providers of healthcare to receive direct feedback from patients and enable them to respond and report back in a way that promotes continual improvement and learning. It is sometimes easier for those outside the organisation to say things that those in it are finding difficult. Checking this out with staff enables them to feel validated in their own experiences and gives them a vehicle in which to raise issues through drawing on the authority of the patient's voice.

Recruiting individuals for the 'right' values

Much has been said about the importance of recruiting staff with the 'right' values. Arguably, courage is one such value. Patterson and colleagues (2014) have identified two theories that focus on the context of employees' values and their impact on the organisation and the workforce.

These are: the 'attraction–selection attrition' theory (Schneider et al., 1995) based on the notion that people over time create a homogenous team as individuals become attracted to those values and thus stay or, if their values are misaligned, leave; and socialisation theory (Cable and Parsons, 2001), when after being recruited, through working closely with others, there is a modification of values as people become 'socialised' into the groups they are working with. However, 'values-based recruitment' is only one component of embedding optimal values in healthcare. Evidence-based recruitment practices such as Situational Judgment Tests (SJTs) allow potential employees to have their values and behaviours tested through exercises that observe their responses to real-life situations that they would face in their role, including coping with pressure and having to challenge a senior on a decision. This, combined with a proper review of the job design, is a far greater predictor of future desired performance than most common recruitment processes. For those who question the potential increased cost of recruitment this needs to be seen against the cost of recruiting someone who becomes overwhelmed or unreasonably disruptive when in post.

Supporting those who 'handle' the emotions

In organisations that are working with emotional material (which is particularly relevant in health and social care), there will always be a need for people who are able to help manage these emotions for the organisation.

The first step is for senior leaders to acknowledge that these people exist, and that they play a vital role, recognising that those with highly developed emotional intelligence are as critical as those with high technical skills. In addition, acknowledgement that emotions will be present and need attending to rather than a culture of just 'sucking it up' will encourage a more healthy processing of emotions which, unless attended to, will show up in a destructive manner either at the individual level (burnout) or organisationally (through disengagement, sabotage or poor performance on the bottom line). Acknowledging the need for this critical role and making space on the organisation's agenda for it to be discussed are critical as is the recognition that if the toxic emotions are due to behaviours of powerful players in the organisation this needs to be handled in a sensitive manner – as seen by Phillippa in Chapter 3.

These 'toxic handlers' need to be identified and nurtured as they often do not ask for help as they are too busy focusing on others (Frost and Robinson, 1999). Building in structures to support them and provide some form of supervision to process their own emotions will prevent them holding on to toxic emotions and burning themselves out. As well as in the everyday supporting of the emotional work of health and social care, these roles will be particularly important at times of organisational change or distress and the level of toxicity they will be processing that is related to wider organisational issues, as opposed to the clinical work, will provide an indicator of the level of comfort with challenge and learning across the organisation (Kilmann, 2011).

Minimising the demands on the toxic handler is important and one that leaders need to pay attention to. Part of doing this is for leaders to be open about the difficulties organisations face and to create opportunities for staff to share their responses and process their emotions. This can be through organisational interventions already discussed (for example, Schwartz Center Rounds®) or by organising large-scale events where staff are invited to discuss how they feel about organisational changes or incidents. We saw this in Chapter 2 when we looked at clinical staff sharing experiences of making mistakes. In their study of organisations and emotional pain, Frost and Robinson (1999) found that executive and middle managers reported this was often the first time they had felt able to talk openly about organisational pain and they themselves were able to express and process their own responses to these issues, making it easier for them to feel comfortable with discussing it with others.

Seeking the view of those outside our own 'group'

Whilst understanding what is happening and why can be found by taking the time to listen to people across the organisation at all different levels; it is also helpful to hear from those outside who interact with us in different ways. This is crucial to overcome groupthink or the 'bandwagon effect', arguably exacerbated through the 'echo-chamber' of social media. Being open to this feedback and hearing it whilst recognising it is only a partial view from their perspective, creating the opportunity for us to think differently about how we are behaving and organising our services and to work collaboratively with others to improve. The key to involving others who are not just outside our organisation but also outside our industry means that we are able to see things from different perspectives.

This requires us to have humility and recognise we have much to learn from others who have different expertise from ourselves. Concepts like 'hackathons' which bring diverse groups of people from different industries and disciplines together to find ways to deal with longstanding issues have led to new ways of delivering services, products and relationships with 'customers'. In its work around experience-based co-design, the Point of Care Foundation is using patients' experiences of services with staff's experiences of trying to provide them, enabling new types of conversation that not only talk about what happened in the interactions but what it felt like for each other. This requires courage on both sides for people to share their emotions and potential vulnerabilities and, at the same time, strengthens the relationship and wider understanding of both the challenges and rewards in healthcare. Staff and patients alike report a re-connection to their work and a sense of greater motivation and enthusiasm to continue to improve.

Developing supporting structures for those who speak up

The biggest concern for any organisation should be when their most passionate people become quiet.

Tim McClure

The impact of individuals displaying moral courage by questioning what is happening, has the potential to promote a collective vitality and virtue; and it can also, initially, result in collective unease, leading to social ostracism and censure of the morally courageous member. This can lead to individuals experiencing disconnection and distress due to condemned isolation (Miller, 1988). In these situations individuals who have spoken out can become anxious about other's reactions and whether further rejection will occur, leading to possible withdrawal – either by leaving, disengaging or becoming inauthentic about their future experiences. Whilst this is clearly distressing and unproductive for the individual, it is also damaging to the organisation as issues that need to be explored no longer get raised, placing greater risk on organisational performance and care. It is therefore important to find ways to offer support to those who do display this type of behaviour.

One way to support people is through the development of training programmes that can help by systematically identifying and addressing some of the individual dimensions of courageous behaviour in employees (such as rationalisation of situations or self-doubt) so that the behaviour becomes more routine (Gentile, 2011), or training people in effective ways of gathering data and evidence to prepare solid cases for their position when raising concerns, thus adopting 'prosocial' behaviour which may be more tolerated by those around them. Much work to date in this area has focused on the lower and middle levels of organisational hierarchy, looking at the identification of corporate or governmental wrongdoing or corruption, or when resisting an organisational policy/strategy to explore how employees might express their disagreement/concern with corporate values and decisions. Yet programmes that focus on specific levels of staff and select cohorts who are similar in their experiences or seniority do not provide for the learning across hierarchies, which often hinder this progress. Helping people to both challenge those in authority and those in authority to be comfortable with being challenged, is fundamental.

Part of being able to muster the courage to act or be is the management of emotions, and learning to control fears and emotions in extreme situations, thus learning to be courageous. Part of this thinking has been adopted in leadership programmes such as the 'Staff College' run by University College Partnership which exposes participants to highly stressful situations to enable them to understand and manage their emotional responses in order to be able to withstand any fearful situation. Clearly this needs to be done sensitively to prevent any excessive stress and subsequent emotional trauma but being able to recognise your own emotional state and manage yourself in a heightened state of arousal is important in an environment such as healthcare.

Maintaining trust with those we strive to serve

Making a mistake, whilst part of being human, in healthcare can have devastating effects. Ask any health professional, and they will tell you their experience with incredible detail even when it may have occurred decades earlier (see Chapter 2).

It requires moral courage to disclose harm caused by error, and what often drives professionals to do this is their overriding concern for their patient. Creating conditions where staff feel an overriding concern for them from their organisations who recognise the difficulty of the work and that mistakes happen will enable staff to feel protected, making it easier for them to act caringly for others and to find the courage they might need to have these difficult, but morally important, conversations.

Insisting that professionals need to be courageous – such as the call from the 6Cs and even the 'Speak up for Safety' campaigns – implies somewhat that conditions of fear, danger or risk are present and that a health professional cannot be ethical without courage. We, however, respectfully disagree with this premise as we believe that whilst good clinical practice requires health professionals to be courageous (as explored in Chapter 2), the managing and organising of healthcare should not.

We need to build settings where courage is rarely needed to do the right thing (these are the 'quantum' organisations described above); ethical work environments are increasingly being shown to provide benefits for patients as well as providers. If health professionals are routinely having to exhibit courage to survive in their practice, this should be a cause for concern not celebration. Courage should not be necessary for any health professional to ask a question or make a suggestion regarding a patient's care. We would go further than that and say that this also applies to patients and their families – as being able to engage in a respectful dialogue shows a level of maturity and shared understanding of the inherent risks in healthcare and a joint endeavour to minimise these risks to keep both the patient and the practitioner safe.

Making 'heroes' of those who behave courageously in relation to their institutions and its hierarchies avoids the question of what is being done to relieve the conditions of potential oppression. Issues such as oppressive conditions, unresponsive systems, bullying clinicians and job insecurity may be tolerated or seen as acceptable in return for those desirable practices of courage, thus feeding the hero's inclination towards moral arrogance and certitude. Celebrating courageous heroes does not shift any wider systemic issues of injustice, abuse of power/position, gender or ethnicity issues, that continue to silence the moral voices of others.

Good healthcare, due to its inherent risk and uncertainty, will always require clinicians to be courageous in their clinical work; it should be acknowledged, nurtured and recognised. The challenge is to look beyond this call for courage to that which focuses on courage in the face of oppressive environments, and to work on diminishing these environments.

Creating productive work spaces

In order to create conditions for courage to flourish, we need to create 'productive workplaces' (Weisboard, 2012). At the core of this principle is getting everyone to improve the whole.

Every approach to change and improvement has its limits, and people will continually be trialling new ones, but what is important is not that you are using the most up to date thinking, but that the approach resonates with the people you are working with – a truism being, 'all models are wrong, some are useful'. We would argue that constantly looking for the 'latest' approach or the 'right' approach and 'what everyone else is doing' is a form of avoidance around taking action or the willingness to have honest conversations about what is really happening locally.

We need to be able to focus our energies on the present. Improving our organisations and societies can be existentially satisfying work, if people avoid the megalomania of believing what you are building will be the final model and all that is needed for the future. Too much time is focused on what will be rather than what is. A constant look to find the latest fad or guru to tell us what to do is ignoring what is. In her work as an organisational development practitioner and executive coach, one of the authors (RM) assists individuals and organisations to confront their reality and their contributions to it. None of us can predict the future and yet people spend so much time thinking about it, ignoring what we can do today. Programmes describing 'new-generation leaders' run the risk of portraying the idea that those currently doing the work are redundant and we have to wait for the next generation to tell us what to do or to save us. This is not courageous but cowardly. It says we cannot do anything and yet all we ever really have is today.

One of the most important things we need is to find the best ways to continually learn together and in a way that people can see the benefit for themselves in doing so.

The learning needs to take place in a space where people feel safe to learn together and do not feel judged for not knowing. All too often, we set up processes that divide our workforce and our customers from each other to learn together. Examples of where people are really learning together and designing together are showing the positive impact of creating more effective care at all levels. But this alone will not create productive workplaces and we need to learn about, and work on, ourselves.

This means that wherever we sit in relation to the 'system', we should find ways to make a positive impact, be it offering our feedback and support to improve things, or listening to others and giving up control and power when it is not in the interest of the whole; this is getting the balance between power and love (Kahane, 2010). This work is about understanding and working on our 'shadow' side, as described at the beginning of this chapter. This is not about a destiny – this is about a life's work.

Finding strategies to make decisions together

In finding ways to help people work together, models and frameworks can be useful. We have seen the introduction of structured, standardised clinical communication tools such as 'SBAR', which enable important information to be communicated rapidly across hierarchical and professional boundaries as a way of enhancing the management of high-risk situations. Other frameworks that attempt to apply logical reasoning to models of communication can also be helpful when trying to bring different groups together to look at complex situations. The physician and philosopher Edward De Bono developed a framework called the 'Six Thinking Hats ®' (De Bono, 1999) which has been more widely adopted in other industries than healthcare but is equally applicable and can be used when working with highly emotive, complex issues and diverse audiences as it provides a structure for the process of decision making.

Figure 6.2   De Bono's 'Six Thinking Hats'

Colour 'hat'	Purpose	Used to
Blue	Process & Control	Structure the thinking
		Identify what needs to be thought about
		Plan actions
White	Fact & Figures	Generate information & data (quantitative & qualitative)
		Create neutrality & objectivity
		Identify the questions to ask

(Continued)

Figure 6.2   (Continued)

Colour 'hat'	Purpose	Used to
Red	Emotions	Get people to share their intuition and hunches
		Surface and explore feelings
		Acknowledge that feelings are important
Green	New Ideas & Creativity	Develop ideas and a range of possibilities
		Provoke different ways of thinking
		Assist in addressing any 'black' hat issues
Yellow	Positive Thinking & Benefits	Identify the positives
		Explore the logic in the ideas
		Share how the ideas are useful
Black	Weaknesses & Risks	Identify the challenges in the ideas including weaknesses and risks

Source: Adapted from De Bono (1999)

The usefulness of this framework is that the process is logical but also values emotional responses and is transparent so it enables participants to ensure all areas to be considered are included and thus increases the likelihood of trusting the outcome.

Creating an environment of reciprocal trust

Whilst we all have a responsibility in creating an environment of trust, the function of the human resources/workforce community is important in how it works with the informal networks that exist in organisations. All too often, the role of HR has become 'to keep the CEO out of court' (Farmer, 2008). Its key role should be about building trust and ensuring that those in senior and powerful positions adopt the principle that employees are basically bright and want to do the right thing, and the only way to relate to people is as intelligent adults. This links back to the work around transactional analysis described in Chapter 2.

Employees can be trusted with bad news as well as good news. They can cope, and an inclusive approach will build confidence, arguing that very few issues that get discussed in the boardroom need to be kept secret from employees (also that the informal networks pick up on them anyway!).

You cannot implement your strategy or test its effectiveness without your staff, so asking them to give views, favourable or not, is critical. Being honest about what you know, and what you do not, and seeking views on how to minimise risk are essential as they are in the interest of the organisation to succeed. It is also important to admit when you have made mistakes and say when you've changed your mind and why. Staff will respect that and see the integrity, but if you do not they will see deceit, which will lead them to no longer trusting you. But whilst senior managers are influential in setting the tone, they are not omnipotent and middle managers and first-line managers are key. The role they play in the translation of not only strategy but also culture is fundamental to organisational success or failure and attention to this is important for both senior leaders and the HR community.

Creating an environment of trust will help us move towards a '*just*' culture (Dekker, 2007). This requires all of us to understand the environment in which people work – context is critical in looking at what contributed to this situation rather than simply who is responsible. Part of this means that judging the actions of others needs to be done by those who understand their work and the conditions in which they are operating. Being clear about what will be helpful in reviewing these situations and agreeing this with all involved is important. If some want retribution whilst others want justification the dialogue will be difficult. Being able to find a shared desired outcome that focuses on healing for all will give us all the best chance of learning and prevention of these issues to others.

By understanding what has happened as an act that is a representation of an organisational, operational, technical, educational, political or cultural issue, then accountability can become forward looking and we can focus on exploring what solutions can be implemented for that problem and who we can involve to implement these improvements and assess if they work.

This shifts people from being the 'problem' to being the source for improvement using an appreciative approach (Cooperider and Whitney, 2005), and offers the possibility of those who have been affected by the action to make a difference for the future. In those cases of relatives of patients 'harmed' by healthcare systems, the individual is at high risk of post-traumatic stress and thus strong social, psychological and organisational support has been shown to reduce the impact of the event and contain some of the negative consequences. For those who have a high internal locus of control, they may well be particularly vulnerable. The benefits of this approach are not just for the individual, but also for the organisation and wider system; in messaging that error is part of the human condition, the effects on all involved can be profound, and that support is available to learn both at an individual and wider system level.

Creating these types of cultures is not an end point, but a continual process which needs to constantly be negotiated by all involved, but by adopting the principles above, it offers the potential to create a more honest and compassionate culture which in itself may lead to more justice in the way errors are responded to, and reduce the fear and thus the need for courage.

Helping staff to enjoy their work

The Institute of Health Improvement has recognised the importance of the environment in which healthcare takes place (Perlo et al., 2017). Whilst not referencing courage specifically, it talks about this in the context of joy in work which impacts on: individual staff engagement and satisfaction; patient experience; quality of care; patient safety; and organisational performance. This acknowledges the current climate in which many staff are working, with reports of burnout, high turnover and low morale. Focusing on enjoying work is helpful because it: moves us to an appreciative frame of inquiry where we look for examples of people enjoying their work and using these experiences to learn from and adopt approaches (Cooperider and Whitney, 2005); often connects us to purpose and meaning and thus in healthcare makes sure that people are able to see how what they do makes a difference to the overall purpose; builds individual and organisational resilience; and enable those who enjoy and get meaning from their work to be more likely to produce better work (Deming, 2000).

To enjoy work people need to feel able to: speak up comfortably; feel physically and psychologically safe; see meaning and purpose in what they do; have a degree of choice and autonomy; feel a sense of *camaraderie* and teamwork; and experience fairness and equality. All of us within healthcare impact on these conditions, irrespective of the different roles we hold, and getting people to understand where they can control or influence the situations they are in and the actions required for change is important. Whilst the research around appreciative inquiry is encouraging, we have seen it misinterpreted as a way of avoiding talking about, or acknowledging, things that are not working well. This not only alienates those whose experiences are not good but also runs the risk of silencing those voices, which in turn risks these issues not being addressed, and deteriorating. Derogatory language such as 'negativity' or laggards used by those advocating positive change are damaging to working with the reality of organisational life and, as in most things, balance is required.

Understanding what needs to be done and who needs to do it, enables organisations to focus their efforts more effectively and also ensures that accountability for change sits in the appropriate place. When thinking about the conditions for people to be able to speak up and what influences that, it is useful to look at organisational structures and see who has the greatest sphere of influence through their interactions with staff, either through direct line management or through their network. The significance of these individuals' behaviours and attitudes to staff speaking out will be critical. Many of these may well be relatively low bands, often people who have moved from being in a senior clinical role to a managerial one and thus not necessarily the most trained or skilled in management. When looking at the NHS staff survey questions such as 'if a friend or relative needed treatment, I would be happy with the standard of care provided by this organisation' or the percentage of staff witnessing potentially harmful errors, near misses or incidents in the last month enables some tracking of these issues but organisations must drill down further than the high level reporting and look at the narrative as well as the figures, if they are to really understand the issues.

'Systems' level

Everything and everyone are connected. Recognising that healthcare organisations do not operate in a vacuum, politicians, regulators, patients and the media need to understand how their behaviour contributes to the conditions that either help or hinder creating the conditions for staff to deliver care. By developing 'intelligent' customer approaches using the ever-expanding knowledge around 'just cultures', safety, 'psychological safety' and 'emotional labour' of work in health and social care and organisational psychology, they can engage in a dialogue which facilitates a more honest and empathic exchange. Greater understanding of how things are interconnected can help connections and relationships between different aspects of life become visible, or reduce 'system blindness' (Oshry, 2007).

We are seeing greater understanding across those in healthcare of 'systems' theory which, whilst helpful, can also 'blind' us to other influences that do not fit into our view of what makes up the 'system'. We are more drawn to what complexity theory (Stacey and Griffin, 2005) has to offer in making sense of what happens in the National Health Service and what contributes to the situations we find ourselves in. We can never fully control the outcome of interventions in 'complex systems' because of the multiple variables that contribute to them and thus we have to continually be paying attention to what our intentions are when making an intervention and monitoring the impact to see if it is assisting us with our overall aim and purpose. The work then becomes about adjusting our own behaviours and assumptions in conjunction with others as the meanings of our actions are defined by the responses of those we are working with. Our intention in writing this book is to promote a more informed dialogue about the role of courage in healthcare and how we can all play our part in supporting each other when we need it, whilst reducing the need for it in raising concerns. Only time will tell, through people's responses to the book, if our intention had the desired outcome. This brings us back to the work above at the individual level around modelling behaviours of inquiry, dialogue and empathy.

We would argue that what we all need from the wider 'system' is less 'independent scrutiny' and more interdependent 'stewardship', slowly but persistently shifting the social norms of holding the NHS and all of us in society, whichever role we play, to account. So what are some of the systemic conditions that reduce the likelihood of people simply following orders from authority figures? These include: closeness to the people affected by our decisions; closeness of those in authority to impact directly on us; whether there is a conflicting view of those in authority; the power and influence of those who are bystanders; and the absence of any sense of personal culpability.

This is particularly relevant when looking at healthcare and the role and relationships with government and Secretaries of State on the following of instructions. Often criticism is made of CEOs and Trust Boards of their reactions to errors or poor performance and their 'bullying' behaviour and yet many staff are unaware of or unsympathetic to the performance measures that CEOs and Boards are subjected to. Stories of 'Monday morning' meetings and phone calls from civil servants in the Department of Health or the Secretary of State when performance is slipping or a critical incident has occurred, are well known in the senior structures of the NHS. A story reported in the *Health Service Journal* of CEOs being asked to chant' 'We can do this', gives some insight into what those seen as the most senior can be subjected to in an environment where performance anxiety is high.

This in turn needs to be seen in the context of how the public respond to their, and their friends and families, own experiences of healthcare and their own sense of responsibility for their own health and the amount of money they are prepared to pay for public services – in the words of the physicist, Fritjof Capra (2016), 'We are all in this together'. Looking at performance in an adversarial environment where 'poor' performance is subject to ritual humiliation, is not conducive to raising concerns, speaking out and engaging in dialogue to deal with the many complex and 'wicked' problems that face the NHS. Despite our desire for simplistic, binary explanations that come down on the position of either 'right' or 'wrong', this situation is perpetuated by the adversarial nature of the debate in the House of Commons (an institution which when originally set up measured the space between the benches of the opposition to government by the length of two swords!), along with reporting from the media at times with the aim of increasing circulation, and playing on the human desire for answers and someone to blame.

The role of the media, and how they portray errors, whilst rightly investigating issues in the public interest, may also be contributing to the overall response to the external environment. In addition, the advent of social media such as Facebook ® and Twitter ®, whilst opening up the debate and sources of stories to wider audiences and greater scrutiny, is difficult for health staff to engage in due to restrictions placed on professionals (be it around patient confidentiality or politically motivated statements), either through their organisational policies or regulatory bodies, and can often make it difficult to give a different perspective on issues which in itself can lead to silencing of different voices and simplification of more complex issues. In professions such as healthcare, the behaviour of the professional regulator is also significant and thus stories of how people are treated by organisations such as the General Medical Council (GMC) or Nursing and Midwifery Council (NMC) will also affect whether people feel able to act in the face of fear. This reference to wider context is key – we often look for people to blame when things go wrong as a way of seeking justice or resolution. The recent case of Bawa Garba, a junior doctor who made a mistake, in what has subsequently been described as a chaotic and understaffed clinical area, is a case in point. An inability to speak up about this at the individual level or to understand it at the organisational/system level means that these situations will continue to repeat themselves.

However, while the ethical arguments are clear, there remains a need for moral courage in disclosing medical errors, especially in an environment that is not open or sensitive to the difficulties in doing so. Threat of professional censure, institutional penalty, malpractice litigation, bad publicity, humiliation and perhaps the perpetuation of the myth of perfectionism in healthcare ('the heroic efforts of the doctors and nurses') all militate against error disclosure. But if the *sine qua non* of our professional ethics is to have regard for the 'other' then the primary question is not whether to disclose but how to in a productive and ethical fashion.

Example from Practice 6.3

Ann, district nurse

Arriving on duty, Ann is given her list with a large number of patients requiring morning insulin. As she is about to set out, her manager takes a call from a colleague who is off sick and so Ann is given a couple of additional patients on an already long list.

She arrives at her third of four patients due, morning insulin, to find that the patient has no more needles which are kept in the patient's home. She checks the patient's blood glucose level and it is 21mmols/l – the patient has a history of hyperglycaemia (often due to diet). She has used her last needle at the first visit of a patient who had also run out and had left some spare to cover them for the evening visit and the next day, having chased her prescription. She rings a colleague who is on the other side of the borough and also hasn't got any as their system has changed and they are now sent to the patient's home directly, thus stock is not kept in the DN stores. She rings the local pharmacist to see if they will issue some for her whilst the new prescription is coming and they refuse without a request from the practice, saying that they are fed up with the GP who isn't sending the scripts through and they aren't getting paid. Ann explains that the patient is hyperglycaemic and offers to get a script at the end of her visits but the pharmacist still refuses. Ann is also conscious that she has another patient waiting for their insulin. She rings the practice and explains and the receptionist says she will need to come and speak to the GP directly and pick up a prescription, as their electronic prescribing isn't working. Ann explains to the patient the situation and that she will return once she has the needles. She has checked all other vital signs and knows the patient is safe and so quickly goes to administer insulin to the other patient and asks if she can take a couple of needles which the patient refuses, saying the nurses often do that. Ann heads back to the practice to see the GP.

Having to wait, when she gets in to to see the GP they are very stressed and irritated with Ann, asking why this situation has arisen. Ann is also annoyed about the situation and plans to pick it up with the nurse who visited the night before and should have seen the situation. The GP then realises the needles are not on repeat prescription, adds this in then prints out the prescription for Ann to take to the pharmacist. Ann leaves the GP to a very full waiting room. Once she has collected the needles she returns to the patient who hands Ann her insulin, which she checks the dosage and the expiry date of and then administers the insulin. On returning to the office Ann writes up her notes and checks the last entry of the person to pick up on the issue of the needles. As she does this she notices that the insulin given is a different type to the one she gave in the morning. She speaks to her colleague who is an HCA who says she doesn't remember but would have given what was prescribed the day before.

(Continued)

(Continued)

Concerned, Ann goes to see the patient to explain what has happened. The incorrect insulin is on the table and the patient tells Ann she has had new medication delivered. When Ann checks the fridge she has two boxes of incorrect insulin. On further inspection there is the latest prescribed insulin at the bottom of the fridge. The patient tells Ann she is confused as the dosage and type keep getting changed between the specialist team and the GP.

Reflections on Ann's experience: When we look at this case we could take the view that Ann was solely responsible for the error, as she should have double-checked the type of insulin. However, when we look at this through the chain of events we can see a number of contributions to this situation, which made the likelihood of error high. A more ethical approach to error disclosure is for the institution or, in this case, wider 'system' to take collective blame for the mistake, recognising the context in which the professionals are working.

Must we be courageous?

We would strongly argue that outside of the courage required to do the 'work' of healthcare, calls for staff to be courageous can suggest an endorsement of an oppressive status quo, diverting attention from the real problems in the culture. The primary goal of healthcare institutions should be about medically excellent and morally good clinical practice.

This is pertinent to evaluating the development of the '6Cs' strategy promoted by the Chief Nursing Officer in response to the Francis Inquiry into standards of care at Mid Staffordshire Hospital. Whilst understanding the significant pressure placed on the CNO and the nursing profession to respond, the positioning of courage as essential to the role of the nurse and other healthcare professionals, speaks to the points above – it begs the question, in a role which is there to provide care and 'protect' or 'advocate' for the patient and their family, why would you need courage to speak out unless the environment in which you work in looks unfavourably on you doing that? Asking clinicians to be courageous in speaking out or up against things they are concerned about suggests this is done in the context of fear – fear of some form of negative retaliation. In which case, the work of us all is to call this out and for those in positions of power and influence to create environments that promote positive cultures where courage is not required. Asking those who are already in a position of distress, be it moral distress due to concerns about clinical practice or emotional distress due to illness or impending mortality, to be courageous in raising concerns, we would argue, is unhelpful.

Valorising courage as essential for good professional practice, and for someone's own good will despite the toll it takes on healthcare, which is inherently risky, should not take place in an environment of organisational fear. Exercising courage is not sufficient to addressing distress in dysfunctional systems and should not be seen as a magic bullet to eliminate moral distress. Actions of individuals will not deal with institutional dynamics, which may well be where the moral distress is operating. If courage is required for people either at junior or senior level to question the way things are done or to speak up for what they believe to be right, conditions of oppression exist (Tessman, 2005). In an environment where oppression exists, the call for courage will be constant and the fear of retaliation or negative consequences for speaking out to prevent harm or maintain integrity, leads to significant stress on those working in those environments. The call for courage deflects attention on the importance of other areas such as knowledge, wisdom, compassion and justice and away from the daily relational call of the work to be fully present with and for others and not distracted by this fear.

Creating the conditions which enable staff, patients and their families to be appropriately courageous, i.e. for their 'role' rather than to speak up about legitimate concerns be they clinical, operational or financial, requires the courage of those in political roles to not be reactive and simplistic in their responses, and the understanding and responsibility of those in the media to explain the complexities and sensitivities of situations when things happen rather than in a sensationalist way just to increase their sales. Part of this is about the NHS being open and honest about the reality of the challenges that are inherent in healthcare. Being able to acknowledge these challenges and then recognise we are all contributing to, and are affected by, them creates the opportunity to engage in more adult-to-adult conversations about how these tensions get managed.

In his work in patient leadership , David Gilbert (2014) speaks about how professionals, in their desire to address power imbalances, talk of 'empowering' patients and lay claim to understanding patients' experience because 'we are all patients'. He rightly challenges them that because of the inherent power, and thus privilege, they hold by being part of a system, saying that they will empower others or 'speak for patients', whilst this may come from positive intent, continues to keep power in their hands. This is not simply a suggestion of professionals and those in leadership roles ceding all their power, as the use of that power in its generative form serves an important function. By the nature of the complexity and political nature of healthcare, the use of legitimate, reward and expert power sources can facilitate opportunities for improvement. We see this below when we look at the interviews with the Secretary of State for Health and Social Care intervening in concerns brought to them by MPs and local constituents or 'activists'.

Courage 'in the moment'

It is 'in the moment' that the ability to balance one's response to the need to be courageous is important. To be able to be reflexive such that you both recognise the force in which you are pushing either love or power, the impact it is having on the overall purpose of creating the conditions for people to be open and honest, and the ability to adjust your behaviour in real time to enable this to occur, is not without its difficulties. We are often driven by the intensity of our feelings such that these two dynamics, rather than in balance, tend to allow one to dominate, making a choice on which to assert. This not only happens at the individual level but is also structural whereby we swing from one position to another rather than take a balanced and often paradoxical view.

In the case of creating the conditions for people to talk about things to improve services, there is a consensus that things need improving but people all have different views on what change is required, often with each believing that the problems would improve if the other changed what they thought or did, and that it is only when stakeholders are prepared to reflect on how they might need to change what they themselves are thinking and doing, that the possibility for improvement comes. Structuring conversations around us all looking at our own contribution to the situation and the impact that has, rather than what others are or are not doing, offers greater promise for positive change. As one of the author's (RM) father would say, 'People are as they are, not as we want them to be'. So if we want to create a social system that enables the difficult work of healthcare to be done in a courageous way and speaking up as just everyday practice, then we need to focus our attention on what *we* are doing to enable that to be a reality rather than wasting energy on trying to change others.

In this recognition of the need for us all to reflect on our own contribution, and what we need to change to create something different, it can be difficult for us to let go of strongly held views, which can keep us stuck. Sometimes this can lead to the need to exclude those who are not willing to embrace new ways of working, which may seem to work against the idea of inclusion and connection but is necessary to address progress. However, doing this without paying attention to power structures creates risk to the overall aim of the work. In the context of healthcare and its emphasis on cure, the power still sits predominantly in key groups: the medical profession, the managerial class and the politicians. The increasing focus on care (due to the increased needs of the older population and their co-morbidity), and the more readily available access to medical knowledge, means that patients and citizens are becoming more vocal and powerful in the way that healthcare is organised and provided. In the context of the workforce roles such as social workers and nurses who have been predominantly focused on care and non-medical influences on health and wellbeing, those are well placed to support this shift if they are willing to step forward into this arena.

Decision making in the NHS, the development of more integrated health and social care, and the increasing role of local councils in healthcare decisions, mean that public scrutiny and the associated accountability are increasing and all contributing to a shift in power.

A political context

You have to learn the rules of the game; then play them better than everyone else.

Albert Einstein

Those wanting to create an environment where error is responded to in a just culture need to know the rules of all parts of the 'game'. This is not about pursuing some Machiavellian ploy or intellectual exercise but about working effectively in the context in which the NHS and a democratic society operate.

Given the level of public money involved in healthcare, it will always have a large political interest. Understanding the political process is important for those working in health to be able to make sense of decisions in the wider context of society. The role the Secretary of State for Health and Social Care plays is important. People in public leadership roles, who have worked with politicians, describe the need for understanding of and empathy for the complexity and pressure of political life, and how those in the system need to work effectively with them (see Irwin Turbitt's work on adaptive leadership at http://www.kafkabrigade.org.uk). In their book, *Glaziers and Window Breakers*, Timmins and Davies (2015) present transcripts of interviews of ten Secretaries of State for Health (SOS), providing a critical insight into their roles and how the environment affects the political process, which in turn affects health policy, and thus the running of the National Health Service. Unfortunately, far too often, the dialogue between those delivering care and those responsible for managing is placed in an adversarial framework, which positions people against each other. The ability to work with those we disagree with is fundamental to effective healthcare, not only by learning to be able to have difficult conversations, as described above, but also to work alongside people you fundamentally disagree with or dislike.

Culture change

If you always do what you've always done, you will always get what you've always gotten.

Henry Ford

Change occurs when one becomes what he is, not when he tries to become what he is not.

Arnold Beisser

If we want to create different conditions for healthcare to be provided, one where the courage to do the work gets recognised and nurtured and one where the raising of concerns and need for improvement become normal everyday practice, we have to be willing to confront where we really are. Cultures are identified through the stories, artefacts, routines and rituals people follow and the way that power is exercised. And whether we like it or not, the dominant view is that speaking up or raising concerns is difficult and leads to poor outcomes. This is because those people who have publicly 'blown' the whistle have been subjected to difficult experiences. We do not doubt that they have had difficult experiences; however, we also know people are raising concerns and challenging the status quo every day in the system but not sharing these experiences, and they do not hit the headlines. A focus on stories where this is happening and the benefits this has brought to organisations and ultimately patient care needs to be amplified across the system. Stories such as those covered throughout the book demonstrate that it can be and is being done. The more this becomes the norm by all of us, for all of us, the better the system we will have.

But it is not just the stories of those who have challenged but also those who have been challenged and how it has helped them that also need to be shared. Sharing how it was the operating department assistant who pointed out to you, the surgeon, the mistake you were about to make and how grateful you are to them for keeping the patient and yourself safe, will encourage others to do the same. Attempting to change culture is a complex and long-term endeavour and, in a complex organisation such as the NHS, particularly challenging as it is not a linear process, but using methods that are inclusive with a clearly articulated vision of what the NHS is trying to achieve and why, is key. Alignment of the desired culture to overall strategy is critical, otherwise a clash of purpose occurs to the frustration of all involved. Asking those 'at the top' of the organisation (or in the case of the NHS those who make decisions about resource allocation) to commit energy and resources to cultural change means they need to see both the relational and transactional benefits in terms of organisational priorities and thus a robust case for change is needed and needs to be able to make sense at the societal, organisational and individual level.

Responding to the fear

Part of being able to facilitate change is to be able to articulate honestly where we are now in a way that resonates with the majority view. Despite the efforts to date to try and create an open and honest culture, people are still fearful and there are few public examples of people displaying the behaviour that in an oppressive culture can be seen as requiring courage. And yet, throughout the book, there are many examples of the everyday practices of staff that are doing that. Amplifying these examples, without diminishing the negative experiences of those seen in Chapter 4, will not only encourage others to follow suit but also help others to learn about how to raise these concerns in a constructive way that serves us all in creating a supportive environment for healthcare.

Working with 'power'

Creating the conditions for enabling people to speak up needs to recognise the role that power plays in either hearing or silencing people's voices. Often an uncomfortable subject, it is important to recognise both the formal and informal power structures that exist and how to either use your own power or draw on the power of others to enable issues to be raised. Greiner and Schein (1989) in their book, *Power and Organisational Development,* explore the importance of understanding and using power in order to be effective in organisations. This is not in any underhand and manipulative way, but as a source of bringing about positive intent.

We often get a sense of where power lies by accident when we try to shift something or act and then experience a negative consequence. Understanding the culture in the organisation in which you work is important and will also give insights into where both the formal and informal power lie. Edgar Schein's (2016) seminal work on culture encourages people to look above and below the surface of organisational life to really understand what happens.

Courage in the collective

As described above, if we want to have the support of creating the conditions for good healthcare, those of us working in it need to appreciate that we need to partner with those outside of it and see ourselves as part of a wider community.

It is helpful to draw on examples of how communities collectively mobilise to take action by using their assets, building bridges with others, including those who are often excluded or marginalised, to improve situations and get organised by building relationships through trust to gain collective power, communion and influence. This requires all of us to understand and value others, direct or indirect experience of an issue; their own context, grievances and contributing factors to their experience. It requires us all to work both within, and around the system, to demonstrate an alternative way without the restrictions of bureaucracy and hierarchy, but without destabilising things at the same time, which over time becomes an accepted norm. Christiansen (2009) suggests four stages of how communities mobilise to form 'social movements' which are not necessarily linear and may have a short or long-term life span depending on the issues that concern them and the progress they make. Christiansen found these movements are often experimenting with alternative and innovative ways to do things and, due often to resource constraints, are creative in finding new ways of achieving things.

Using this approach can help to challenge the 'system' and nudge those in formal roles to be open to new ways of working. As well as informing those 'outside' about the constraints in which those in the 'system' work, this sharing can lend itself to ways of tackling this together – creating more 'human' institutions as well as more authentic relationships between statutory organisations and their communities (del Castillo et al., 2016). The NHS England 'Health as a social movement' programme builds on the approach established in the Five Year Forward View (published October 2014), to support social movements in health and care (see www.england.nhs.uk/new-care-models/vanguards/empowering/social-movement). The programme aims to identify and develop exemplar social movements, demonstrate 'what works' and support spread and adoption.

Conclusion

Although how to create these conditions is not new, our ability to draw on the knowledge and expertise of those from the social sciences has been limited by our lack of attention to these experts. Dominated by the positivism model of science – which privileges the subjective and biological sciences over the social – it is interesting to note that quality improvement and organisational development theory has been known about and used in industry for many years and the evidence around safety well researched by organisational psychologists such as Professor Charles Vincent since 1985. If we are truly to create the conditions for courage to both flourish and no longer be required, we would suggest that all of us need to pay attention to our own and collective opinions, and listen to the voices of others, many of whose expertise and experience are greater than our own.

In their research around highly reliable organisations, the Agency for Healthcare Research and Quality recognises that in services such as healthcare we are working in complex, high-hazard domains and that safety is not a static feature but emergent, requiring constant attention and adjustment to risk. One of the key features that they identify in highly reliable organisations is deference to expertise. In creating conditions in which courage is required to provide the care but not for raising concerns and reporting errors, it is a reminder to us all that the evidence exists – we just need to pay attention to it however uncomfortable it might be.

Finally, it is important to remember that this is an iterative process that doesn't stop; each generation needs to be educated as to the risks and the strategies to overcome them, be it at the individual, group, organisational or 'system level' as we have shown, because we all contribute. So if we want a healthcare service that is one where people speak up when concerned and lessons are learnt when errors are made, and we don't want to repeat the mistakes of the past, we need to individually and collectively 'be the difference that makes the difference'.

Useful Weblinks

www.kingsfund.org.uk/publications/what-does-public-think-about-nhs
www.pulsetoday.co.uk/political/political-news/jeremy-hunt-receives-patient-safety-award/20036231.article

https://uthscsa.edu/gme/documents/Circles.pdf
www.nesta.org.uk/sites/default/files/learning_to_take_risks_learning_to_succeed.pdf
www.kingsfund.org.uk/blog/2018/01/how-can-nhs-tap-innovations-front-line
www.telegraph.co.uk/news/health/news/9242893/Hospital-handwashing-campaign-was-exceptionally-successful.html
www.careopinion.org.uk
www.forbes.com/sites/quora/2018/02/28/are-you-in-a-social-media-echo-chamber-how-to-take-an-objective-look/#6c60611561f9
www.hsj.co.uk/workforce/nhs-leaders-chant-we-can-do-this-at-aande-improvement-summit/7020633.article

References

Bakan, D. (1966) *The Duality of Human Existence: An Essay on Psychology and Religion.* Chicago, IL: Rand McNally.

Bancroft-Turner, D. (2008) *Workplace Politics Pocket Book.* Alresford, Hampshire: Management Pocketbooks Ltd.

Berne, E. (1964) *Games People Play – The Psychology of Human Relationship.* Harmondsworth: Penguin.

Bion, W.R. (1998) *Experiences in Groups.* New York: Routledge.

Bowlby, J. (1988) *A Secure Base: Parent–Child Attachment and Healthy Human Development.* New York: Basic Books.

Britnell, M. (2015) *In Search of the Perfect Health System.* New York: Palgrave.

Brown, B. (2017) *Braving the Wilderness: The Quest for True Belonging and the Courage to Stand Alone.* London: Vermilion.

Cable, D.M. and Parsons, C.K. (2001) 'Socialization tactics and person–organization fit', *Personnel Psychology,* 54(1): 1–23.

Capra, F. (2016) *We Are All In This Together.* Available at http://www.fritjofcapra.net

Chaleff, I. (2015) *Intelligent Disobedience: Doing Right When What You're Told To Do Is Wrong.* San Francisco, CA: Berrett-Koehler Publishers.

Christiansen, J. (2009) *Four Stages of Social Movements,* EBSCO Research Starters.

Clegg, C., Bolton, L., Offutt, R. and Davis, M. (2014) *Work Design for Compassionate Care and Patient Safety. Implementing Culture Change within the NHS: Contributions from Occupational Psychology.* London: British Psychological Society.

Cook, A.F. and Hoas, H. (2008) 'Ethics and rural healthcare: What really happens? What might help?', *American Journal of Bioethics,* 8(4): 52–56.

Cooperider, D. and Whitney, D. (2005) *Appreciative Inquiry: A Positive Revolution in Change.* San Francisco, CA: Berrett-Koehler Publishers.

Covey, S.R. (1999) *The 7 Habits of Highly Effective People.* New York, NY: Simon and Schuster.

Davies, H.T.O. and Nutley, S.M. (2000) 'Developing learning organisations in the new NHS', *British Medical Journal,* 320(7240): 998–1001.

De Bono, E. (1999) *Six Thinking Hats.* Harmondsworth: Penguin Books.

Dekker, S. (2007) *Just Culture: Balancing Safety and Accountability.* Farnham: Ashgate.

Del Castillo, J., Khan, H., Nicholas, L. and Finnis, A. (2016) *Health as a Social Movement: The Power of People in Movements.* London: Nesta.

Deming, W.E. (2000) *Out of the Crisis.* Cambridge, MA: MIT Press.

Farmer, N. (2008) *The Invisible Organisation: How Informal Networks can Lead Organisational Change*. Farnham: Routledge.

Frost, P.J. and Robinson, S.L. (1999) 'The toxic handler: Organizational hero and casualty', *Harvard Business Review*, 77(4): 96–106.

Garratt, B. (2010) *The Fish Rots From the Head: The Crisis in our Boardrooms – Developing the Crucial Skills of the Competent Director*. London: Profile Books.

Gentile, M.C. (2011). 'Giving voice to values: Building moral competence' in D .R. Comer and G. Vega (eds), *Moral Courage in Organizations: Doing the Right Thing at Work*. Armonk: M.E. Sharpe, pp. 117–129.

Gergen, K. (1999). *An Invitation to Social Constructionism*. London: Sage.

Gilbert, D. (2014) 'We are all Patients. Yes and No', *Future Patient* [blog]. Available at: https://futurepatientblog.com/2014/11/28/we-are-all-patients-yes-and-no (accessed 12 June 2018).

Greiner, L.E and Schein, V.E. (1989) *Power and Organisational Development – Mobilising Power to Implement Change*. Reading, MA: Addison Wesley Publishing Company.

Guha, N. (2018) *How Can the NHS Tap into Innovations from the Front Line?*, The King's Fund, 16 January [blog]. Available at: www.kingsfund.org.uk/blog/2018/01/how-can-nhs-tap-innovations-front-line (accessed 11 June 2018).

Hamric, A.B, Arras, J.D and Mohrmann, M. (2015) 'Must we be courageous?', *Hastings Center Report*, 45(3): 33–40.

Janis, I.L (1982) *Groupthink: Psychological Studies of Policy Decisions and Fiascos* (2nd edn). Boston, MA: Houghton Mifflin.

Kahane, A. (2010) *Power and Love: A Theory and Practice of Social Change*. San Francisco, CA: Berrett-Koehler Publishers Inc.

Kidder, R. (2006) *Moral Courage*. New York, NY: Harper Collins.

Kilmann, R. (2011) *Quantum Organizations: A New Paradigm for Achieving Organizational Success and Personal Meaning*. Newport Coast, CA: Kilmann Diagnostics.

Kilmann, R.. O'Hara, L. and Strauss, J. (2011) *Organizational Courage Assessment*. Newport Coast, CA: Kilmann Diagnostics.

Kline, R. (2014) 'The "snowy white peaks" of the NHS: A survey of discrimination in governance and leadership and the potential impact on patient care in London and England', Middlesex University's Research Repository. Available at: www.england.nhs.uk/wp-content/uploads/2014/08/edc7-0514.pdf (accessed 12 June 2018).

Miller, J.B. (1988) 'Connections, disconnections, and violations', *Work in Progress*, No. 33. Wellesley, MA: Stone Center Working Paper Series.

Oshry, B. (2007) *Seeing Systems: Unlocking the Mysteries of Organizational Life*. San Francisco, CA: Berrett-Koehler Publishers.

Patterson, F., Zibarras, L. and Edwards, H. (2014) *Values-based Recruitment for Patient Centred Care Implementing Culture Change within the NHS: Contributions from Occupational Psychology*. London: British Psychological Society.

Perlo, J., Balik, B., Swensen, S., Kabcenell, A., Landsman, J. and Feeley, D. (2017) *IHI Framework for Improving Joy in Work*, IHI White Paper. Cambridge, MA: Institute for Healthcare Improvement.

Rolfe, H. (2010) *Learning to Take Risks, Learning to Succeed*. London: National Institute of Economic and Social Research.

Schein, E. (2013) *Humble Inquiry: The Gentle Art of Asking Instead of Telling*. San Francisco, CA: Berrett-Koehler Publishers.

Schein, E. (2016) *Organizational Culture and Leadership* (5th edn). New York: Wiley.

Schneider, B., Goldstein, H.W. and Smith, D.B. (1995) 'The ASA framework: An update', *Personnel Psychology*, 48(4): 747–773.

Stacey, R.D. and Griffin, D. (2005) *A Complexity Perspective on Researching Organisations*. London: Taylor & Francis.

Tessman, L. (2005) *Burdened Virtues: Virtue Ethics for Liberatory Struggles*. Oxford: Oxford University Press.

Tillich, P. (1954) *Love, Power and Justice: Ontological Analyses and Ethical Applications*. New York: Oxford University Press.

Timmins, N. and Davies, E. (2015) *Glaziers and Window Breakers: The Role of the Secretary of State for Health in their own Words*. London: The Health Foundation.

Turbitt, I. http://www.kafkabrigade.org.uk

Turnball, J.E. (2001) 'A systems approach to error reduction in health care', *Japan Medical Association Journal*, 44(9): 392–403.

Weisboard, M. (2012) *Productive Workplaces Revisited: Dignity, Meaning and Community in the 21st Century* (3rd edn). New York: John Wiley & Sons.

West, M. and Dawson, J. (2012) *Employee Engagement and NHS Performance*. London: The King's Fund. Available at: www.kingsfund.org.uk/sites/default/files/employee-engagement-nhs-performance-west-dawson-leadership-review2012-paper.pdf (accessed 13 June 2018).

West, M.A. and Markiewicz, L. (2004) *Building Team-based Working: A Practical Guide to Organizational Transformation*. Malden, MA: Blackwell Publishing.

West, M., Alimo-Metcalfe, B., Dawson, J., El Ansari, W., Glasby, J., Hardy, G., et al, (2012) *Effectiveness of Multi-Professional Team Working (MPTW) in Mental Health Care: Final Report*. NIHR Service Delivery and Organisation Programme.

Williams, S., Michie, S. and Patani, S. (1999) *Improving the Health of the NHS Workforce*. London: Nuffield Trust.

World Health Organisation (WHO) (2012). Patient Safety Research: A Guide for Developing Training Programmes. Available at: http://apps.who.int/iris/bitstream/handle/10665/75359/9789241503440_eng.pdf;jsessionid=AB0D48567D39C3B2A6FD0CD0239EDF35?sequence=1

WHO Surgical Safety Checklist (2009) Available at: http://www.who.int/patientsafety/safe-surgery/checklist/en

Wren, B. (2016) *The Tales of Organisational Life: Using Psychology to Create New Spaces and Have New Conversations at Work*. London: Karnac Books.

FINAL THOUGHTS

We believe that courage takes place in a relational context and is actually a function of an individual, group or wider systemic environment.

Courage is, of course, at the risk of a paralysis by analysis, even from simply defining it. This book has tried not to settle on a definitive definition of courage, though it appears to us that courage is a quality needed by professionals and patients alike when facing situations that leave us feeling vulnerable and fearful and in navigating the emotional tenacity effective healthcare can require. Intuitively, it seems that all clinicians, practitioners, patients and service users, need some courage, but the question of the *need* for courage in healthcare becomes much subtler and more complex the more you look at the nature of courage in healthcare.

Is the need for courage inevitable to practise medicine and provide health*care*? We would argue, *Yes*.

Should we accept the ever-present need for courage in challenging each other and the 'system' when seeking to improve the conditions for those using the healthcare system and those working in it? We would argue, *No*.

Is courage in healthcare a necessary virtue or a warning sign?

Thank you.

Shibley Rahman and Rebecca Myers
London, April 2018

INDEX

Note: Page numbers in *italics* indicate figures.